222 Pecan Candy Recipes

(222 Pecan Candy Recipes - Volume 1)

Cindy Taylor

Copyright: Published in the United States by Cindy Taylor/ © CINDY TAYLOR

Published on November, 28 2020

All rights reserved. No part of this publication may be reproduced, stored in retrieval system, copied in any form or by any means, electronic, mechanical, photocopying, recording or otherwise transmitted without written permission from the publisher. Please do not participate in or encourage piracy of this material in any way. You must not circulate this book in any format. CINDY TAYLOR does not control or direct users' actions and is not responsible for the information or content shared, harm and/or actions of the book readers.

In accordance with the U.S. Copyright Act of 1976, the scanning, uploading and electronic sharing of any part of this book without the permission of the publisher constitute unlawful piracy and theft of the author's intellectual property. If you would like to use material from the book (other than just simply for reviewing the book), prior permission must be obtained by contacting the author at author@papayarecipes.com

Thank you for your support of the author's rights.

Content

222 AWESOME PECAN CANDY RECIPES 6

1. Addicting Chocolate Pecan Saltine Delights Recipe 6
2. Arkansas Millionaires Recipe 6
3. Aunt Bills Brown Candy Recipe 6
4. Auntie Karens Nuk U Lar Fudge Recipe 7
5. BUTTERY MIXED NUT BRITTLE Recipe 7
6. Best Ever Peanut Brittle Recipe 7
7. Bevs Never Fails Micro Fudge Recipe 8
8. Bourbon Balls Recipe 8
9. Bourbon Pecan Balls Recipe 9
10. Brandy Balls Recipe 9
11. Bull Dog Brittle Recipe 9
12. Butter Pecan Fudge Recipe 9
13. Buttermilk Candy Recipe 10
14. Buttermilk Pecan Pralines Recipe 10
15. Butterscotch Fudge Recipe 10
16. Butterscotch Nut Fudge Recipe 11
17. COCONUT PECAN CLUSTERS Recipe 11
18. Canadian Chocolate Fruit Roll Recipe 11
19. Candied Apples Recipe 12
20. Candy Pecan Roll Dated 1962 Recipe 12
21. Candy Strawberries Recipe 12
22. Cappuccino Caramels Royale Recipe........ 13
23. Caramel Brownies Recipe 13
24. Caramel Chocolate Rolo Pretzels Recipe.. 13
25. Caramel Fudge Recipe 14
26. Caramel Kisses Recipe 14
27. Caramel Nut Candy Recipe 15
28. Caramels Recipe 15
29. Chattanooga Chew Chews Recipe 16
30. Cheese Candy Recipe 16
31. Cherry Nut Easter Eggs Recipe 16
32. Chocolare Cherry Snowballs Recipe 17
33. Chocolate Billionaires Recipe 17
34. Chocolate Bourbon Truffles Recipe 17
35. Chocolate Butter Crunch Toffee Recipe ... 18
36. Chocolate Cappuccino Candy Recipe 18
37. Chocolate Caramel Graham Crackers Recipe 18
38. Chocolate Cherries Recipe 19
39. Chocolate Cherry Pistachio Fudge Recipe 19
40. Chocolate Coated Coconut Balls Recipe 20
41. Chocolate Cream Cheese Fudge Recipe 20
42. Chocolate Crunch Recipe 21
43. Chocolate Dipped Apricots Recipe 21
44. Chocolate Dreams Recipe 21
45. Chocolate Fudge Squares Recipe 22
46. Chocolate Pecan Brittle Recipe 22
47. Chocolate Pecan Candy Recipe 22
48. Chocolate Pecan Toffee Recipe 23
49. Chocolate Truffles 23
50. Chocolate Truffles Recipe 23
51. Chocolate Turtle Bars Recipe 24
52. Chocolate Butterscotch Pecan Fudge Ala Easy Recipe 24
53. Chocolate Coconut Truffles Recipe 25
54. Cobblestone Candy Recipe 25
55. Coconut Pecan Clusters Recipe 25
56. Cornflake Candy Recipe 26
57. Cracker Candy Recipe 26
58. Cranberry Candy Recipe 26
59. Cranberry Coconut Fruit Balls Recipe....... 27
60. Cranberry Fudge Recipe 27
61. Cranberry Nut Chocolate Bark Recipe 27
62. Cranberry Nut Fudge Recipe 28
63. Cream Candy Recipe 28
64. Cream Cheese Fudge Recipe 28
65. Creme Divinity Kraft Foods Marshmallow Cream Recipe 29
66. Creole Candy Recipe 29
67. Creole Creamy Pecan Pralines Recipe 30
68. Creole Orange Flavored Pecans Recipe 30
69. Dark Chocolate ButterCrunch Recipe 30
70. Dark Chocolate Cococans Recipe 31
71. Date Drops Recipe 31
72. Delicious Homemade Creme Filled Chocolate Candy Recipe 32
73. Divine Divinity Recipe 32
74. Double Nut English Toffee Recipe 33
75. Double Nut English Toffee Recipe Recipe 33
76. Dr Pepper Pralines Recipe 34
77. Dressed Up Chocolate Bark Recipe 34
78. Easy Apricot Balls Recipe 35
79. Easy Chocolate Fudge Recipe 35
80. Easy Chocolate Macaroons Recipe 35
81. Easy Delicious Nutty Marshmallow Log

	Recipe 36	
82.	Easy Microwave Pralines Recipe 36	
83.	Easy Peanut Butter Chocolate Fudge Recipe 36	
84.	Easy Peanut Butter Fudge 37	
85.	Easy Toffee Recipe 37	
86.	Elegant Marshmallows Recipe 38	
87.	Elegant Martha Washington Candy Recipe 38	
88.	English Toffee Recipe 39	
89.	Extravagant Old Fashioned Fudge Dated 1942 Recipe 39	
90.	Fudge Recipe 39	
91.	Graham Break Aways Recipe 40	
92.	Graham Cracker Brittle Recipe 40	
93.	Graham Cracker Nut Brittle Recipe 41	
94.	Graham Cracker Snacks Recipe 41	
95.	Heirloom Cream Candy Recipe 41	
96.	Holiday Candy Fudge Bars Recipe 41	
97.	Homemade Cinnamon Praline Pecans Recipe 42	
98.	Honey Macadamia Nut Fudge Recipe 42	
99.	I Forgot To Make The Fudge Recipe 43	
100.	Inside Out Caramel Apples Recipe 43	
101.	Louisiana Pralines Recipe 44	
102.	Macadamia Cashew Crunch Recipe 44	
103.	Maple Pecan Fudge Recipe 45	
104.	Marilyns Rocky Road Heaven Recipe 45	
105.	Marshmallow Nut Truffles Recipe 46	
106.	Martha Washington Balls Recipe 47	
107.	Mexican Orange Candy Recipe 47	
108.	Mexican Pralines Recipe 47	
109.	Microwave Fudge Recipe 48	
110.	Microwave Praline Recipe 48	
111.	Microwave Pralines 1 Recipe 48	
112.	Microwave Sugar Spiced Pecans Recipe ... 49	
113.	Microwave Toffee Recipe 49	
114.	Millionaires Recipe 49	
115.	Missouri Colonels Recipe 50	
116.	Moms Secret Fudge Recipe Recipe 50	
117.	My Favorite Fudge Recipe 51	
118.	My Favorite Fudge Recipe 51	
119.	My First Chocolate Fudge Recipe 52	
120.	My Homemade Toffee Recipe 52	
121.	My Tutti Frutti Fudge Recipe 52	
122.	NUTTY SWEET CARAMELS Recipe 53	
123.	New Orleans Pralines Recipe 54	

124.	No Bake Cocoa Bourbon Balls Recipe 54
125.	Nutty Caramels Recipe 54
126.	Nutty Heavenly Hash Recipe 54
127.	Old Fashion Brown Sugar Fudge Recipe .. 55
128.	Old Fashioned Date Confection Recipe ... 55
129.	Orange Chocolate Meltaways Recipe 55
130.	Orange Juice Balls Recipe 56
131.	Orange Pecans Recipe 56
132.	PECAN CLUSTERS Recipe 56
133.	PECAN DELIGHTS Recipe 57
134.	POOR MAN TURTLES Recipe 57
135.	PRETZEL BITES Recipe 57
136.	Pa & Ma's Wonderful Holiday Fudge Recipe 58
137.	Peanut Brittle Wanda Recipe 58
138.	Peanut Brittle Ice Cream Pie With Chocolate Sauce Recipe 58
139.	Peanut Buttery Chocolate Balls Recipe 59
140.	Pecan Caramel Spiders Recipe 59
141.	Pecan Caramel Spiders Recipe 60
142.	Pecan Brittle Recipe 62
143.	Pecan Clusters Recipe 62
144.	Pecan Diamonds From The Culinary Institute Of America Recipe 62
145.	Pecan Divinity Recipe 63
146.	Pecan Molasses Brittle Recipe 63
147.	Pecan Penuche Recipe 64
148.	Pecan Pralines Recipe 64
149.	Pecan Roll Recipe 64
150.	Pecan White Chocolate Brownies 65
151.	Pecan Chocolate Chip Cookie Brittle Recipe 65
152.	Poor Mans Millionaires Recipe 66
153.	Poppycock Recipe 66
154.	Positively Yummy Pumpkin Fudge Recipe 66
155.	Praline Grahams Recipe 67
156.	Praline Pecans Recipe 67
157.	Pralines Anyone Recipe 67
158.	Pralines Recipe 68
159.	Pralines With Pecans Recipe 68
160.	Pronto Pralines Recipe 68
161.	Pumpkin Fudge Recipe 69
162.	Pumpkin Pie Fudge Recipe 69
163.	Quick Nut Fudge Recipe 70
164.	ROLLO PRETZELS Recipe 70
165.	Raisin Cashew Chocolate Fudge Recipe 70

166. Red Pepper Fudge Recipe 71
167. Reindeer Nibbles Recipe 71
168. Rich Creamy Pistachio Tangerine Fudge Recipe 72
169. Rocky Road Balls Recipe 72
170. Rocky Road Fudge Recipe 73
171. Rolo Pretzel Turtles Recipe 73
172. Rose Water And Ginger Poached Pears With Caramel Glaze On A Bed Of Crunch Vanilla Cream Recipe 73
173. Rum Balls Recipe 74
174. Rum Raisin Fudge Recipe 75
175. SOUTHERN PRALINES Recipe 75
176. SPIRIT BALLS Recipe 75
177. Saltine Toffee Cookies Recipe 76
178. Salty Chocolate Pecan Candy Recipe 76
179. Salty Sweet Treat Recipe 76
180. Seaside Candy Rolls Recipe 77
181. Sees Fudge The Best Recipe 77
182. Simple Yummies Recipe 78
183. Some Kinda Rich Fudge Dated 1964 Recipe 78
184. Spiced Nuts Recipe 79
185. Spiced Pumpkin Fudge Recipe 79
186. Sugar Cookie Chocolate Crunch Fudge Recipe 79
187. Sugar Free Chocolate Fudge Recipe 80
188. Sugared Nuts Delight Recipe 80
189. Swedish Candied Nuts Recipe 81
190. Sweet Autumn Spiced Pecans Recipe 81
191. Sweet Spiced Fancy Nuts Recipe 82
192. Sweet Swedish Pecans Recipe 82
193. THREE CHOCOLATE FUDGE WITH PECANS Recipe 82
194. Texas Millionaire Candy Recipe 83
195. Texas Style Microwave Pralines Recipe 83
196. The Best Christmas Fudge Recipe 84
197. The Delta Queen's Pralines Recipe 84
198. Toffee Recipe 84
199. Traditional Buttermilk Pralines Recipe 85
200. Trevor City Fudge Recipe 85
201. Triple Chocolate Sour Cherry Fudge Recipe 85
202. Triple Nut Candy Recipe 86
203. Triple Nut Toffee Recipe 86
204. Turtle Squares Recipe 86
205. Turtles Recipe 87

206. Vanilla Fudge With Pecans Recipe 87
207. Wanda Riggs Fudge Recipe 88
208. Whipped Fudge Recipe 88
209. White Bark Candy Recipe 89
210. White Chocolate And Eggnog Fudge Recipe 89
211. White Chocolate Truffles Recipe 90
212. White Fudge Recipe 90
213. White Popcorn Balls Recipe 91
214. White Or Chocolate Eggnog Fudge Recipe 91
215. Wicked Kahlua Fudge Recipe 91
216. Yummy Buttermilk Candy Recipe 92
217. Devinity Candy Recipe 92
218. Microwave Pralines Recipe 92
219. Pecan Bark Recipe 93
220. Pina Coloda Bonbons Recipe 93
221. Super Easy Cream Cheese Rum Fudge Recipe 93
222. Velveeta Cheese Fudge Recipe 94

INDEX 95
CONCLUSION 97

222 Awesome Pecan Candy Recipes

***

1. Addicting Chocolate Pecan Saltine Delights Recipe

Serving: 24 | Prep: | Cook: 10mins | Ready in:

Ingredients

- 24 saltine crackers
- 1 cup light brown sugar
- 1/2 cup unsalted butter
- 6 ounces chocolate chips
- 1/2 cup chopped pecans

Direction

- Lay saltines side by side on a cookie sheet.
- Heat brown sugar and butter until dissolved then pour over saltines and bake at 450 for 5 minutes.
- Cover with chocolate chips and spread.
- Sprinkle with pecans and allow to sit at room temperature for at least an hour.

2. Arkansas Millionaires Recipe

Serving: 10 | Prep: | Cook: 10mins | Ready in:

Ingredients

- 1 pkg kraft caramels
- 2 cups broken pecans
- 1/2 block paraffin
- 2 to 3 tablespoons milk
- 1 large package of milk chocolate chips

Direction

- Melt caramels and milk in top of double boiler.
- Beat for 3 minutes.
- Add pecans and drop on buttered platter or waxed paper.
- Melt choc chips and paraffin or even a little less paraffin.
- Dip caramel nut drops in mixture and cool on wax paper.

3. Aunt Bills Brown Candy Recipe

Serving: 30 | Prep: | Cook: 30mins | Ready in:

Ingredients

- 3 cups sugar, divided
- 1 cup half and half
- 1/4 cup water
- 1/4 teaspoon baking soda
- 5 tablespoons unsalted butter, cut into cubes
- 1/2 teaspoon vanilla extract
- 1 pound pecans, toasted, coarsely chopped (about 4 cups)

Direction

- Butter 8x8x2-inch metal baking pan. Combine 2 cups sugar and half and half in heavy large saucepan. Stir occasionally over low heat until sugar dissolves. Set aside.
- Bring remaining 1 cup sugar and 1/4 cup water to boil in heavy medium saucepan over medium-low heat, stirring until sugar dissolves. Increase heat; continue boiling without stirring until syrup turns deep amber, brushing sides of pan with wet brush and swirling pan, about 8 minutes.
- Immediately pour caramel syrup into half and half mixture in large saucepan (mixture will bubble). Stir constantly over medium-low heat until caramel dissolves. Attach candy thermometer to side of pan. Increase heat to

medium. Continue cooking and stirring until mixture registers 244°F, about 12 minutes. Remove from heat and immediately stir in baking soda (mixture will foam slightly). Add butter and stir to melt. Let stand without stirring until mixture cools to 160°F, about 20 minutes. Mix in vanilla. Using large wooden spoon, stir constantly until candy begins to thicken and loses its gloss, 4 to 5 minutes. Mix in nuts (candy will be very stiff). Scrape candy into prepared pan. Using wet fingertips, press candy firmly into pan. Cool completely, then cut into 30 squares

4. Auntie Karens Nuk U Lar Fudge Recipe

Serving: 36 | Prep: | Cook: 1mins | Ready in:

Ingredients

- 1 12 oz. bag milk or dark chocolate chips
- 1/2 cup semi-sweet chocolate chips
- 1 can sweetened condensed milk
- 1 teaspoon vanilla
- 1 cup chopped pecans

Direction

- Combine all chips, condensed milk and vanilla in a microwave-safe bowl.
- Nuke on high 1 minute, stirring at 30 seconds.
- Continue to cook in 10-15 second bursts until the chocolate completely melts when beaten.
- Add nuts and beat until smooth and fudgy; pour in 8x8-inch square pan lined with wax paper. Chill until set; cut into squares and serve.

5. BUTTERY MIXED NUT BRITTLE Recipe

Serving: 24 | Prep: | Cook: 60mins | Ready in:

Ingredients

- 2 cups sugar
- 1 cup light corn syrup
- 1/2 cup water
- 1 cup butter, cut into bits
- 4 cups mixed raw nuts (I use walnuts, almonds, pecans and pine nuts)
- 2 tsp. vanilla extract
- 1/1-2 tsp. baking soda
- Non-stick spray

Direction

- Spray two baking sheets and set aside.
- In a large heavy saucepan, mix sugar, corn syrup and water.
- Cover and heat to boiling over medium heat.
- Add butter, stir until butter is melted.
- Insert candy thermometer.
- Over medium heat, cook without stirring until the mixture reaches 305 degrees (35 – 45 minutes)
- Gradually add nuts, keeping mixture boiling.
- Remove from heat.
- Add vanilla and baking soda. Beat vigorously 15 seconds, being careful not to splatter.
- Immediately pour onto the two baking sheets. Spread evenly with two forks, until thin and fairly even thickness.
- Cool completely.
- Break into pieces.
- Store in airtight container (I refrigerate it)

6. Best Ever Peanut Brittle Recipe

Serving: 12 | Prep: | Cook: 10mins | Ready in:

Ingredients

- 2 cups sugar
- 1/2 cup water
- 1 stick unsalted butter
- 1/3 cup light corn syrup
- 1/2 teaspoon baking soda
- 12 ounces roasted salted peanuts, cashews, pistachios and/or pecans
- Fleur de sel or crushed Maldon sea salt

Direction

- Prep does not include cooling of recipe.
- In a large saucepan, combine the sugar, water, butter and corn syrup and bring to a boil.
- Cook over moderately high heat, stirring occasionally, until the caramel is light brown and registers 300° on a candy thermometer, 10 minutes.
- Remove from the heat and carefully stir in the baking soda. The mixture will bubble.
- Stir in the nuts, then immediately scrape the brittle onto a large rimmed, non-stick baking sheet.
- Using the back of a large spoon (oil it lightly if it sticks), spread the brittle into a thin, even layer.
- Sprinkle with salt. Let cool completely, about 30 minutes.
- Break the brittle into large shards.
- Make Ahead The brittle can be stored in an airtight container at room temperature for up to 1 month

7. Bevs Never Fails Micro Fudge Recipe

Serving: 15 | Prep: | Cook: 18mins | Ready in:

Ingredients

- 3 cups sugar
- 3/4 cup butter
- 5 oz. can evaporated milk
- 1 (12 oz.) bag of chocolate chips
- 10 oz. jar of marshmallow creme
- 1 cup chopped pecans or walnuts
- 1 tsp. vanilla
- Because quantity sizes of things have changed since I first cre
- ated this you may need to use different size can and jars of evap. milk and marshmallow creme.

Direction

- Combine sugar, butter and evaporated milk in large buttered glass (3 quart or larger) bowl. Cover with plastic wrap.
- Microwave 10 minutes on medium high
- Stir
- Recover and micro another 8 minutes - should now be at soft ball stage but micros vary
- Fold in marshmallow crème, nuts, and vanilla
- Fold in fast because it sets up very quickly
- Pour into 9 x 13 inch pan
- Chill
- Cut into squares

8. Bourbon Balls Recipe

Serving: 12 | Prep: | Cook: | Ready in:

Ingredients

- 3 cups vanilla wafers, rolled to powder consistancy
- 3 Tbsp corn syrup
- 1 cup confectioners' sugar
- 1/2 cup cocoa powder
- 1 cup very finely chopped pecans
- 1/2 tsp vanilla extract
- 1/2 cup bourbon

Direction

- Mix all ingredients together.
- Roll into small 3/4 inch balls.
- Roll balls in confectioners' sugar, cocoa or shredded coconut.
- Makes about 3 dozen.

9. Bourbon Pecan Balls Recipe

Serving: 16 | Prep: | Cook: | Ready in:

Ingredients

- 2 cups whole pecans
- 1 cup graham cracker crumbs
- 1/2 cup confectioner's sugar
- 2 ounces bourbon
- 2 tablespoons light corn syrup

Direction

- Coarsely chop 1 cup pecans and reserve.
- Grind remaining pecans then combine with crumbs, sugar, bourbon and corn syrup.
- Using buttered hands form into balls and roll in chopped nuts.

10. Brandy Balls Recipe

Serving: 24 | Prep: | Cook: | Ready in:

Ingredients

- 3 cups vanilla wafers finely crushed
- 2 cups powdered sugar
- 1 cup pecans finely chopped
- 1/4 cup cocoa
- 1/2 cup brandy
- 1/4 cup light corn syrup
- powdered sugar

Direction

- Mix crushed wafers, powdered sugar, pecans and cocoa.
- Stir in brandy and corn syrup then shape mixture into 1" balls and roll in sugar.
- Cover tightly and refrigerate several days.

11. Bull Dog Brittle Recipe

Serving: 20 | Prep: | Cook: 12mins | Ready in:

Ingredients

- 8 graham crackers
- 1 stick butter
- 1/2 cup sugar
- 1 cup chopped pecans

Direction

- Line 15 x 10 inch cookie sheet with foil.
- Lay graham crackers on foil leaving space between each cracker.
- Sprinkle nuts over crackers.
- Melt butter. Add sugar. Stir constantly.
- Bring to a boil and boil for 2 minutes. Pour over nuts.
- Bake at 350 degrees for 10 to 12 minutes. DO NOT LET BROWN!!

12. Butter Pecan Fudge Recipe

Serving: 36 | Prep: | Cook: | Ready in:

Ingredients

- 1 2/3 cup brown sugar, firmly packed
- 2/3 cup evaporated milk
- 2 cups mini marshmallows
- 1 1/2 cups butterscotch chips
- 1 cup toasted pecans, chopped
- 1 tsp. vanilla

Direction

- Combine sugar and milk in saucepan.
- Heat to boiling. Boil 5 minutes stirring constantly.
- Mixture will appear curdled.
- Remove from heat and add marshmallows, chips, nuts and vanilla.

- Stir until marshmallows and chips melt.
- Pour into buttered 9x9 pan.
- Chill and cut into squares.

13. Buttermilk Candy Recipe

Serving: 0 | Prep: | Cook: | Ready in:

Ingredients

- 2 cups sugar
- 1 cup buttermilk
- 1/4 cup butter
- 1/2 tsp soda
- 2 TBS corn syrup
- pecans
- 1 tsp vanilla

Direction

- Mix (minus the vanilla) and heat over medium heat in a large pot until it comes to a boil and thickens. Set off heat and add vanilla. When lukewarm, beat until thick as for fudge. Pour out into buttered plate. This candy turns a rich brown before your eyes.

14. Buttermilk Pecan Pralines Recipe

Serving: 810 | Prep: | Cook: 40mins | Ready in:

Ingredients

- 1 cup buttermilk
- 2 cups sugar
- Large pinch salt
- 1 teaspoon baking soda
- 2 teaspoons vanilla
- 1/8 pound butter (1/2 stick, or 4 tablespoons)
- 2 cups pecans

Direction

- Stir the buttermilk and sugar together plus soda and salt, and cook in deep pot, stirring all the time until mahogany brown in color. Add vanilla, butter and beat till almost thick. Add nuts and drop by spoonful on marble slab or parchment paper to cool.

15. Butterscotch Fudge Recipe

Serving: 16 | Prep: | Cook: 10mins | Ready in:

Ingredients

- 1c firmly packed dark brown sugar
- 1(7.5oz.)jar marshmallow Fluff
- 2/3c evaporated milk
- 6Tbs unsalted butter
- 1/2tsp salt
- 1(12oz)bag white chocolate chips
- 2c chopped almonds,pecans or walnuts
- 1tsp vanilla extract

Direction

- Line an 8" square baking pan with heavy duty foil, leaving a 1" overhang on 2 sides.
- In a heavy medium saucepan, combine brown sugar, marshmallow fluff, milk, butter and salt and bring to a boil over med-high heat. Reduce heat to medium and simmer, stirring constantly with wooden spoon, for 5 mins. Remove pan from heat, add white chocolate chips and stir till melted. Blend in nuts and vanilla.
- Scrape fudge into prepared pan. Refrigerate till firm, 2-3 hours.
- Remove fudge from pan, using foil to lift it out. Then cut into 16 cubes, serve. Or chill in an airtight container for up to a week.

16. Butterscotch Nut Fudge Recipe

Serving: 24 | Prep: | Cook: 5mins | Ready in:

Ingredients

- 1-3/4 cups sugar
- 1 jar (7 oz.) marshmallow creme
- 3/4 cup evaporated milk
- 1/4 cup (1/2 stick) butter
- 1-3/4 cups (11-oz. pkg.) HERSHEY'S butterscotch chips
- 1 cup chopped salted mixed nuts or pecans
- 1 teaspoon vanilla extract

Direction

- Line 8-inch square pan with foil, extending foil over edges of pan.
- Combine sugar, marshmallow crème, evaporated milk and butter in heavy 3-quart saucepan.
- Cook over medium heat, stirring constantly, until mixture comes to full boil; boil and stir 5 minutes.
- Remove from heat; gradually add butterscotch chips, stirring until chips are melted.
- Stir in nuts and vanilla.
- Pour into prepared pan; cool.
- Refrigerate 2 to 3 hours.
- Remove from pan; place on cutting board.
- Peel off foil.
- Cut into squares.
- Store tightly covered in refrigerator.
- About 5 dozen pieces or about 2-1/4 pounds candy.
- NOTE: For best results, do not double this recipe.

17. COCONUT PECAN CLUSTERS Recipe

Serving: 10 | Prep: | Cook: 15mins | Ready in:

Ingredients

- 1 1/2 C. pecan pieces
- 1 C. flake coconut
- 8 oz. of almond bark (white or chocolate)

Direction

- Toast pecan pieces in the microwave 1-2 min.
- Melt almond bark according to the package directions.
- Mix coconut and pecans into melted Almond bark & drop by teaspoon onto wax paper and let harden.

18. Canadian Chocolate Fruit Roll Recipe

Serving: 8 | Prep: | Cook: 5mins | Ready in:

Ingredients

- 3/4 lb semi sweet chocolate chips
- 1/4 cup sugar
- 2 oz butter
- 1/2 cup chocolate cookie crumbs
- 1 1/2 cups chopped dried fruit
- 1/2 cup chopped asorted nuts (walnuts, pecans, almonds setc)
- 3/4 cup raisins

Direction

- Melt chocolate with butter and sugar.
- Blend in all remaining ingredients.
- Spread mixture flat on parchment paper.
- Shape mixture into a cylinder using the parchment to help roll it.
- Chill well.
- When well chilled, slice and serve along with pound cake, strawberries and cream.

19. Candied Apples Recipe

Serving: 10 | Prep: | Cook: 45mins | Ready in:

Ingredients

- 3 lbs apples (I used Granny Smith green apples)
- 1 pkg (16oz) chocolate candiquik
- 1 pkg (16oz) vanilla candiquik
- Individually wrapped caramels (50 pieces) (+2 T water)
- Wooden dowels or lollipop sticks
- Crushed pecans, almonds, M&M's, or any candy you wish!

Direction

- Melt the whole package of caramels with 2 Tbsp. water over low to medium-low heat, stirring constantly.
- I started by dipping the apples in caramel and placing back on the wax paper to cool – to speed up the process, place them in the fridge to cool.
- Once the apples have cooled and the caramel is set, melt both flavors of CANDIQUIK according to the directions on the package and dip away - coating as much or little of the apple as you wish.
- And the rest is up to you to get as creative as you like!
- Enjoy...they are delicious!

20. Candy Pecan Roll Dated 1962 Recipe

Serving: 16 | Prep: | Cook: 20mins | Ready in:

Ingredients

- 1 cup granulated sugar
- 1 cup brown sugar
- 2 tablespoon corn syrup
- 2/3 cup milk
- 1/4 teaspoon salt
- 2 tablespoons butter
- 1 teaspoon vanilla
- 1/2 cup finely chopped pecans

Direction

- In 2 quart saucepan mix sugar, milk, corn syrup and salt.
- Cook over medium heat stirring constantly until sugar is dissolved.
- Cook stirring occasionally to 234 degrees on candy thermometer.
- Remove from heat and add butter.
- Cool mixture to 120 without stirring.
- Add vanilla.
- Beat vigorously for 10 minutes with wooden spoon.
- Shape candy into 12-inch roll.
- Roll in 1/2 cup finely chopped pecans.
- Wrap and chill until firm.
- Cut into slices.

21. Candy Strawberries Recipe

Serving: 16 | Prep: | Cook: | Ready in:

Ingredients

- 2 (3 oz.) pkgs. strawberry gelatin
- 1 c. flaked coconut
- 1 c. chopped pecans
- 3/4 c. Eagle Brand milk
- 1/2 tsp. vanilla
- Red decorators sugar

Direction

- Mix gelatine, coconut and pecans.
- Stir in vanilla and milk.
- Mix well.
- Chill in refrigerator for 1 hour.
- Shape into small balls or into the shape of strawberries.
- Roll in red sugar.

22. Cappuccino Caramels Royale Recipe

Serving: 64 | Prep: | Cook: 15mins | Ready in:

Ingredients

- 1 cup (2 sticks) butter or margarine
  2 (1-ounce) squares unsweetened chocolate, cut up   2 1/4 cups firmly packed brown sugar   1 (14-ounce) can EAGLE BRAND sweetened condensed milk (NOT evaporated milk)
  1 cup light corn syrup
  1 tablespoon instant coffee crystals
  1 cup chopped pecans or walnuts (optional)

Direction

- Line 8-inch square baking pan with foil, extending foil over edges of pan. Butter foil; set aside
- In heavy 3-quart saucepan, melt butter and chocolate. Stir in brown sugar, EAGLE BRAND, corn syrup and coffee crystals. Clip candy thermometer to side of pan. Cook over medium heat, stirring constantly, until thermometer registers 248 (firm-ball stage*). Mixture should boil at moderate, steady rate over entire surface. (It should take 15 to 20 minutes to reach firm-ball stage)
- Remove from heat. Remove thermometer. Immediately stir in nuts (optional)
- Remove from heat. Remove thermometer. Immediately stir in nuts (optional). Quickly pour into prepared pan, spreading evenly with spoon. Cool
- When candy is firm, use foil to lift candy out of pan. Use buttered knife to cut into squares. Wrap each square in plastic wrap or place in candy cups if desired

23. Caramel Brownies Recipe

Serving: 24 | Prep: | Cook: 15mins | Ready in:

Ingredients

- 1 (18.25 ounce) package German chocolate cake mix with pudding
- 3/4 cup melted butter
- 1/3 cup evaporated milk
- 1 cup chopped pecans
- 13 ounces individually wrapped caramels, unwrapped
- 1/3 cup evaporated milk
- 1 cup semi-sweet chocolate chips

Direction

- Preheat oven to 350 degrees F (175 degrees C). Spray one 9x13 inch pan with non-stick coating.
- Combine the cake mix, butter and 1/3 cup evaporated milk. Mix well and pour 2/3 of the batter into pan.
- Press pecans into batter and bake for 8 to 10 minutes.
- In a saucepan over medium heat, combine the caramel and 1/3 cup evaporated milk. Stir until melted and smooth; pour over cooled cake mix.
- Sprinkle chocolate chips on top of caramel and top with spoonfuls of remaining cake mix. Bake for additional 15 to 18 minutes; cool and cut.

24. Caramel Chocolate Rolo Pretzels Recipe

Serving: 48 | Prep: | Cook: 20mins | Ready in:

Ingredients

- 48 Rold Gold Classic Twist pretzels
- 48 Rolo caramel Chocolate candies (unwrapped)

- 48 pecan halves

Direction

- Preheat oven to 275.
- On a cookie sheet spread out 3 rows of 4 pretzels about 2 inches apart.
- Place Rolo candy in center of pretzel.
- Put on lowest rack of oven for around 8-10 minutes.
- DO NOT let candy completely melt flat. You ONLY want it softened.
- Remove cookie sheet from oven and smoosh 1 pecan into the center of the Rolo candy.
- Place back in oven and bake just long enough to roast the pecan around another 8-10 minutes.
- Allow to cool and then remove and place in an airtight container.
- They won't last long!

25. Caramel Fudge Recipe

Serving: 78 | Prep: | Cook: | Ready in:

Ingredients

- 6 c sugar, divided
- 2 c light cream
- 1/4 t baking soda
- 1/2 c butter or margarine
- 8 1/2 c (2 lbs.) pecans, broken

Direction

- The flavor of this golden brown fudge comes from the caramelized sugar. Combine 4 cups sugar and cream in a heavy 4-quart saucepan. Set aside. Melt 2 cups sugar in a heavy 10-inch skillet over medium heat. Stir sugar constantly until it begins to melt. Heat sugar-cream mixture over medium heat. Continue melting sugar in skillet, stirring and watching closely so it does not scorch. As soon as it is completely melted, pour liquid sugar in a thin stream into boiling sugar-cream mixture, stirring constantly. Do not let sugar remain over heat after completely melted; this will produced a scorched taste. Cook combined mixtures to 246 degrees F. Remove from heat and add baking soda and butter. Stir in and let candy stand for 30 minutes. Add nuts. Stir to mix; pour into buttered 9-inch square pans. Cool slightly and cut into squares. Makes about 78 pieces.

26. Caramel Kisses Recipe

Serving: 20 | Prep: | Cook: 20mins | Ready in:

Ingredients

- Waxed paper or deep baking trays
- butter
- 4-5 cups chopped pecans
- 2 cups sugar
- 1 cup light Karo or other corn syrup
- 1/4 tsp salt
- 16 oz. cream

Direction

- Spread several sheets of waxed paper on table or cabinet; butter the paper, then sprinkle pecans over it. Or butter the baking trays and sprinkle nuts in them. (You'll need more nuts for the waxed paper method.)
- Mix sugar, syrup, salt, and half of cream. Stir mixture until it boils then turn down heat.
- Add remainder of cream and cook slowly, stirring constantly, until mixture forms a firm ball in cool water.
- Pour mixture over pecans in trays, or on waxed paper.
- Cover with more waxed paper, if using.
- Cool completely and cut into pieces.

27. Caramel Nut Candy Recipe

Serving: 12 | Prep: | Cook: 10mins | Ready in:

Ingredients

- 1 large bag of wrapped caramels (or 2)
- 2 cups chopped walnuts, pecans
- 2 Tbs. cream, heavy or regular whipping cream
- 1 Tb. butter with salt
- (Optional-2-3 cups finely chopped walnuts, pecans or peanuts. You can also roll in toasted or untoasted coconut.)
- **You can toss in a handful or two of chocolate chips, too!

Direction

- The prep time is as long as it takes to unwrap all those caramels. Children love to help do this so keep an extra bag around just in case they eat some before you use them in the recipe.
- I use about 30-50 of them, depending on my pan size. If you use a 9x13 pan, use about 30 caramels.
- Unwrap your caramels and put them in a microwave-proof glass bowl with the cream and butter. Microwave on high until the caramels lose their gloss and can be stirred easily. You can stir the caramels every two minutes during the cooking process.
- After the caramels have melted, stir the mixture well, blending in the butter and cream. Add the nuts and stir well.
- Pour the entire mixture into a pan and let the mixture cool and set completely which depending on your kitchen's temperature, may take up to an hour or more.
- To cut the caramels, run a knife under hot water and dry off then cut the caramels into small squares.
- IF YOU WANT TO MAKE A NUT ROLL, before the caramel sets and is still warm to the touch, you can cut out rectangles of any length desired, and using buttered hands, roll the warm caramel into the nuts or coconut as mentioned above in the optional additions suggested under the list of ingredients. Slice rolls of this candy with toasted coconut on the outside make a lovely presentation.

28. Caramels Recipe

Serving: 64 | Prep: | Cook: 30mins | Ready in:

Ingredients

- 2 c. sugar
- 1/2 c. butter
- 2 c. whipping (heavy) cream
- 3/4 c. light corn syrup
- additional butter, for pan
- --------------------
- Flavor Options:
- (You can use one, all, or none)
- 1/2 c. chopped pecans
- 1 tsp. vanilla
- sea salt

Direction

- Grease bottom and sides of square pan, 8 x 8 x 2 or 9 x 9 x 2 inches, with additional butter. Spread pecans in pan, if using.
- Heat 1/2 cup butter, sugar, cream, and corn syrup to boiling in 3-quart heavy saucepan over medium heat, stirring constantly. Cook, stirring frequently, to 245 degrees F on candy thermometer or until small amount of mixture dropped into very cold water forms a firm ball that holds its shape until pressed.
- Remove from heat and add vanilla, if using, stirring rapidly to incorporate. Immediately pour into pan (over pecans, if using); cool.
- If desired, sprinkle tops of caramels with small amount of sea salt - you would not believe how delicious this is.
- Cut into 1-inch squares. Wrap individually in plastic wrap or waxed paper.

29. Chattanooga Chew Chews Recipe

Serving: 32 | Prep: | Cook: 25mins | Ready in:

Ingredients

- Crust: 2 cups all purpose flour
- 1 cup brown sugar
- 1 cup pecans, chopped
- 1/2 cup salted butter (NO SUBSTITUTES)
- caramel topping : 1 cup butter
- 3/4 cup brown sugar 1 (12 oz. package semi-sweet chocolate

Direction

- Preheat oven to 350 degrees F.
- In bowl mix flour, butter, and brown sugar. Press into ungreased 9x13-inch pan. Sprinkle pecans evenly over unbaked crust.
- For caramel topping: Melt brown sugar and butter in a saucepan. Bring to a boil and continue to boil for 1 min., stirring constantly.
- Pour caramel mixture over crust and pecans. Bake for 20-25 min. or until surface is bubby.
- Remove from oven sprinkle chocolate chips over hot surface. Gently swirl melted chocolate chips with a spatula for a marbled effect.
- Cool at least 5 hours. Cut into small squares (very rich candy!)

30. Cheese Candy Recipe

Serving: 12 | Prep: | Cook: 10mins | Ready in:

Ingredients

- 1 8 oz cream cheese
- 2 cups chopped pecans
- 1 box sifted powdered sugar
- 1 teaspoon vanilla

Direction

- Toast pecans lightly.
- Melt cream cheese in a double boiler; add powdered sugar, vanilla and pecans.
- Drop by spoonfuls onto waxed paper.

31. Cherry Nut Easter Eggs Recipe

Serving: 8 | Prep: | Cook: 15mins | Ready in:

Ingredients

- 1/2 c. milk
- 1/2 stick butter
- 2 (3-oz.) pkgs. vanilla pudding and pie filling (not instant)
- 9-oz. jar maraschino cherries
- 1 c. finely chopped pecans or walnuts
- 1 to 2 lbs. confectioners' sugar
- 1 lb. chocolate, melted

Direction

- Cut cherries in half, and drain well on paper towels.
- Cook milk, butter and pudding in a medium saucepan on low heat until well blended and thick. Remove from stove and add cherries, nuts and enough sugar to make a thick consistency.
- Form the mixture into 8 to 10 egg shapes with hands coated in butter. Place on wax paper covered cookie sheet. Chill several hours until firm.
- Melt chocolate being careful not to scorch it. Frost egg with melted chocolate. Decorate with butter cream icing.

32. Chocolare Cherry Snowballs Recipe

Serving: 0 | Prep: | Cook: 1hours | Ready in:

Ingredients

- 1 -9oz package chocolate cookie wafers, finely crushed (about 2-1/4 c)
- 1-1/2 cups dried cherries, coarsely chopped
- 1 cup flaked coconut
- 1 cup pecans, chopped and toasted
- 1- 14oz can sweetened condensed milk
- 1 tsp vanilla
- powdered sugar or unsweetened cocoa powder

Direction

- In large bowl, stir together all ingredients except powdered sugar or cocoa powder. Cover bowl, refrigerate until firm (about 3 hours).
- Form rounded teaspoonfuls into 1-inch balls.
- Sprinkle balls with powdered sugar or cocoa.
- Place on waxed paper, store in fridge.

33. Chocolate Billionaires Recipe

Serving: 28 | Prep: | Cook: 5mins | Ready in:

Ingredients

- 1- package caramels unwrapped (about 14 ounces)
- 3- tablespoons water
- 1 1/2 - cups of chopped pecans
- 1- cup crisp rice cereal....like (Rice Krispies)
- 3- cups milk chocolate chips
- 1 1/2 - teaspoons shortening

Direction

- Line 2 baking sheets with waxed paper, grease the paper and set aside.
- In a large heavy saucepan, combine the caramels and water, cook and stir over low heat until smooth.
- Stir in pecans and rice cereal until all is coated.
- Drop by teaspoonsfuls onto prepared pans.
- Refrigerate for 10 minutes or until firm.
- Meanwhile melt chocolate chips and shortening, stir until smooth.
- Dip candy into chocolate coating entire candy and place back onto waxed paper.
- Refrigerate until set.
- Then store in airtight containers.
- Yields approx. 2 pounds.

34. Chocolate Bourbon Truffles Recipe

Serving: 26 | Prep: | Cook: 15mins | Ready in:

Ingredients

- 1 can (14 ounces) sweetened condensed milk
- 3 cups semisweet chocolate chips
- 1 Tablespoon vanilla extract
- 2 Tablespoons bourbon (if you don't like bourbon you can substitute it with Frangelico, Bailey's Irish Creme, Kahlua coffee liqueur, Cointreau, Grand Marnier, creme de menthe or any other liqueur.)
- 1/2 to 3/4 cup pecans, finely chopped
- granulated sugar, unsweetened cocoa, or very finely chopped pecans

Direction

- Combine chocolate chips and sweetened condensed milk in a saucepan over low heat.
- Heat, stirring, until melted and smooth.
- Remove from heat.
- Stir in the vanilla, bourbon, and 1/2 to 3/4 cup pecans.
- Transfer to a small bowl.
- Cover and chill for 3 to 4 hours, or until mixture is firm.

- Working with fingertips, shape into 1-inch balls.
- Roll in finely chopped pecans, sugar, coconut or unsweetened cocoa.
- Place on a tray or baking sheet, cover loosely, and chill for at least 1 hour.
- If desired, put each truffle in a decorative fluted paper or foil cup and keep in tightly covered container in the refrigerator until giving or serving.
- Keep these refrigerated, tightly covered.

35. Chocolate Butter Crunch Toffee Recipe

Serving: 8 | Prep: | Cook: 20mins | Ready in:

Ingredients

- 1/2 pound unsalted butter
- 1 cup granulated sugar
- 3 teaspoons water
- 1 teaspoon vanilla
- 8 small milk chocolate bars
- 1 cup chopped pecans

Direction

- Stir butter, sugar and water well and bring to rapid boil stirring constantly.
- Remove from fire and add vanilla then pour into shallow buttered pan.
- Place chocolate bars on top and spread with spatula.
- Sprinkle with pecan then cool and break into pieces.

36. Chocolate Cappuccino Candy Recipe

Serving: 0 | Prep: | Cook: 15mins | Ready in:

Ingredients

- 1 TBSP. instant coffee granules.... get a good coffee
- 1 TBSP. hot water
- 2 cups sugar
- 1 cup evaporated milk
- 1/2 cup butter
- 1 (12-ounce) bag of semisweet chocolate morsels
- 1 (7-ounce) jar marshmallow cream
- 1 cup chopped pecans
- 1 TBSP. finely grated orange rind
- 2 teasp. orange or orange extract
- 2 teasp. brandy extract

Direction

- Combine the coffee granules and the water.
- Stir until the granules are dissolved. Set aside.
- Combine the sugar, milk, and butter in a large saucepan.
- Cook over medium heat until mixture comes to a boil, stirring constantly.
- Boil 10 minutes, stirring constantly. Remove from heat after the 10 minutes.
- Add chocolate morsels and the marshmallow cream. Stirring until melted.
- Stir in coffee mixture, pecans, orange rind and the orange and brandy extracts. Mix well.
- Spread mixture evenly in a well-buttered 13 x 9 x 2-inch pan.
- Cover and chill.
- Cut into squares.
- Store in refrigerator.
- Yields: 2 3/4 pounds

37. Chocolate Caramel Graham Crackers Recipe

Serving: 30 | Prep: | Cook: 15mins | Ready in:

Ingredients

- 12 (4 3/4- by 2 1/2-inch) graham crackers

- 1-1/2 sticks (3/4 cup) unsalted butter, cut into pieces
- 1/2 cup packed light brown sugar
- 1/8 teaspoon salt
- 1 -1/2 cups semisweet chocolate chips (9 1/2 oz)
- 1 cup walnuts, pecans, or almonds (3 to 4 oz), toasted and chopped

Direction

- Preheat oven to 375°F.
- Line a 15- by 10- by 1-inch baking pan with foil, leaving a 2-inch overhang at each end.
- Line bottom of pan with graham crackers (it will be a tight fit).
- Melt butter in a 1 1/2- to 2-quart heavy saucepan over moderately low heat, then add brown sugar and salt and cook, whisking, until mixture is smooth and combined well, about 1 minute.
- Pour butter/sugar mixture over crackers, spreading evenly.
- Bake in middle of oven until golden brown and bubbling, about 10 minutes.
- Scatter chocolate chips evenly over crackers and bake in oven until chocolate is soft, about 1 minute.
- Remove pan from oven and gently spread chocolate evenly over crackers with offset spatula.
- Sprinkle nuts evenly over chocolate and cool crackers in pan on a rack 30 minutes.
- Freeze until chocolate is firm, 10 to 15 minutes.
- Carefully lift crackers from pan by grasping both ends of foil, then peel foil from crackers. Break crackers into serving pieces.
- Cooks' note:
- • Crackers keep, chilled and layered between sheets of wax paper in an airtight container, 2 weeks.

38. Chocolate Cherries Recipe

Serving: 15 | Prep: | Cook: 5mins | Ready in:

Ingredients

- 1 - 7 1/4 oz pk vanilla wafers, finely crushed
- 1/2 c powdered sugar
- 1/2 c pecans
- 1/4 c boiling water
- 1 T margarine
- 1 T corn syrup
- 2 t instant coffee
- 30 maraschino cherries with stems
- 3 - 6 oz pk semi-sweet morsels

Direction

- Mix vanilla wafers, powdered sugar and nuts.
- Combine water, margarine, corn syrup and coffee.
- Add to vanilla wafer mixture.
- Shape approximately 1/2 tablespoon of this mixture around each cherry.
- Cover and refrigerate 2 hours.
- Melt and stir chocolate over low heat approximately 5 minutes until melted.
- Hold stems and dip cherries in chocolate coating carefully and completely.
- Refrigerate.
- Note:
- May be prepared ahead of time.

39. Chocolate Cherry Pistachio Fudge Recipe

Serving: 30 | Prep: | Cook: | Ready in:

Ingredients

- 1 ½ cups granulated sugar
- 1 cup evaporated milk
- 2 T butter
- ¼ tsp fleur de sel
- 2 cups marshmallows

- 2 oz 85% cocoa chocolate, chopped
- 8 oz bittersweet chocolate, chopped
- ¼ cup pistachios, chopped
- ¼ cup pecans, chopped
- ½ cup dried cherries

Direction

- Line and 8 inch square baking pan with foil.
- Combine sugar, evaporated milk, butter and salt in a medium, heavy bottomed saucepan. Bring to a full rolling boil over medium heat, stirring constantly. Boil, stirring constantly, for 5-6 minutes. Remove from heat.
- Stir in everything that's leftover until marshmallows and chocolate are melted. Pour into prepared baking pan. Refrigerate for 2 hours or until firm. Lift from pan, remove foil, cut into pieces.
- Stores well in wax paper in a zip lock.

40. Chocolate Coated Coconut Balls Recipe

Serving: 40 | Prep: | Cook: 60mins | Ready in:

Ingredients

- 1 can (14-15 oz.) sweetened condensed milk (NOT evaporated milk)
- 1 stick butter or good quality margarine
- 1 teaspoon vanilla extract
- 2 1 lbs boxes confectioners sugar
- 15 - 16 oz. flaked coconut
- 2 cups chopped pecans
- 12 oz. package semi-sweet chocolate chips
- 1 block Gulf paraffin wax

Direction

- Mix milk, butter and vanilla.
- Add confectioners' sugar.
- Then add pecans and coconut. Mix well. (It will be necessary to mix with washed hands as mixture maybe quite stiff)
- Chill 15 minutes.
- Form into balls the size of walnuts and insert a tooth pick in center of each ball.
- Chill again.
- Melt chocolate chips and paraffin wax in top of double boiler.
- Remove from heat.
- Dip each candy ball in chocolate.
- Remove quickly and place on wax paper.
- Use a spoon dipped in chocolate to smooth over hole left from toothpick.
- Refrigerate candy balls.
- Enjoy!

41. Chocolate Cream Cheese Fudge Recipe

Serving: 14 | Prep: | Cook: 20mins | Ready in:

Ingredients

- 4 squares unsweetened chocolate
- 8 oz. cream cheese
- 4 cups confectioners' sugar
- 1-1/2 tsps. vanilla extract
- Note: Instead of vanilla extract I add liqueur ie. Baileys or Frangelico or whatever.
- 1/2 cup pecans or walnuts, chopped

Direction

- Melt chocolate in microwave, then cool to room temperature.
- With cream cheese at room temperature, mix cream cheese with melted chocolate.
- Add confectioners' sugar and vanilla extract.
- Pour into an 8 x 8 inch pan.
- Refrigerate for a couple of hours before cutting.
- If you want to add a peanut butter flavour, add 1/2 cup peanut butter and increase sugar to 5 cups.

42. Chocolate Crunch Recipe

Serving: 16 | Prep: | Cook: | Ready in:

Ingredients

- 4 ounces milk chocolate
- 4 ounces white chocolate
- 1 stick butter
- 1/2 cup whipping cream
- 1 cup chopped pecans
- 2/3 cup chopped dates
- 1/2 pound ladyfingers coarsely crushed

Direction

- Line bottom of a round cake pan with parchment paper then butter or spray with baking spray.
- Break chocolate into small pieces.
- Place milk chocolate in one bowl and white chocolate in another.
- Add 4 tablespoons butter to each.
- Stand bowls over pans of hot water until chocolate and butter have melted stirring occasionally.
- Place bowls on counter and stir half the cream, nuts, dates and crushed cookies into each.
- Spoon darker chocolate mixture into pan and spread level with back of a spoon.
- Push mixture down into the corners then top with white chocolate mixture.
- Cover with foil or plastic wrap and chill until set.
- Remove from pan and serve cut into slices.

43. Chocolate Dipped Apricots Recipe

Serving: 24 | Prep: | Cook: 15mins | Ready in:

Ingredients

- 1/2 cup sugar
- 1-1/2 cups water
- 1 lb. dried apricots
- 4 ounces bittersweet chocolate, coarsely chopped (or semisweet)
- 1 tablespoon chopped pecans

Direction

- Line a cookie sheet with parchment paper and put a wire rack on top.
- Combine sugar and water in a small saucepan; bring to a boil, stirring to dissolve the sugar. Reduce the heat to medium and simmer for 3 minutes. Add apricots and gently simmer 5 minutes. Transfer the apricots with a slotted spoon to the rack. Let cool completely. They should not be wet when dipping them.
- Melt chocolate in a double boiler of simmering water. Dip half of a poached apricot in the chocolate, letting excess drip off. Sprinkle with chopped pecans over the chocolate half and return the apricot to the rack. Repeat with the remaining apricots. (You will have some melted chocolate left over.) Refrigerate until the chocolate has set, about 20 minutes.

44. Chocolate Dreams Recipe

Serving: 15 | Prep: | Cook: 5mins | Ready in:

Ingredients

- 2 cups sugar
- 1/4 cup butter
- 1 teaspoon vanilla
- 1 cup chucky peanut butter
- 1 cup chopped pecans
- 14 large marshmellows
- 1/2 cup milk
- 1/4 cup cocoa
- 1/8 teaspoon salt

Direction

- Mix sugar, milk and butter in a medium size saucepan.

- Boil, stirring constantly, for 1 minute.
- Add remaining ingredients; stir well.
- Drop by teaspoon onto waxed paper or pour into a buttered pan and cut into bars when cooled.

45. Chocolate Fudge Squares Recipe

Serving: 10 | Prep: | Cook: 20mins | Ready in:

Ingredients

- 360g of real good dark chocolate
- 1 cup of condensed milk
- 2/3 cup of walnuts or pecan nuts crushed, but not powdered

Direction

- Break chocolate in small pieces (or buy chocolate buttons) and melt them in a ban-marie set.
- After the chocolate is melted, pour in the condensed milk (continue to cook in ban-marie). Stir together until the mixture is thick enough so you can see the bottom of the bowl (or pan). Just tilt the bowl, if it's ready, the mixture will no longer stick to the bowl. This happens very quickly.
- Remove the bowl (or pan) from the bain-marie and add the walnuts or pecans. The nuts should be crushed to small pieces, but not too much so they become a powder. Mix to combine. Reserve. Let it cool a bit.
- Wash a terrine with water, but don't dry it with a cloth. Cover the interior of the terrine with Clingfilm leaving some hanging out so you can fold it in. Pour the mixture in the terrine, press it down to make an even and smooth surface. Fold the hanging Clingfilm to cover the fudge.
- Leave it in the refrigerator until it sets. Cut it into small squares and serve. You can dust the bars with cocoa powder if you prefer a bitter taste.

46. Chocolate Pecan Brittle Recipe

Serving: 10 | Prep: | Cook: 20mins | Ready in:

Ingredients

- 2 cups butter
- 2 cups sugar
- 1/4 cup plus 2 tablespoons water
- 12 ounces milk chocolate candy bars
- 3 cups chopped pecans

Direction

- Combine butter, sugar and water in a large saucepan then cook over low heat until mixture reaches hard crack stage.
- Remove from heat and immediately pour into 2 buttered pizza pans spreading to edges of pan.
- Melt chocolate and spread over brittle then sprinkle pecans evenly on top and press into chocolate.
- Let stand until chocolate is firm and break into pieces.

47. Chocolate Pecan Candy Recipe

Serving: 1 | Prep: | Cook: 5mins | Ready in:

Ingredients

- 4-1/2 cups sugar
- 12 oz. can evaporated milk
- 1 cup butter or margarine
- 3 cups (18 oz) semisweet chocolate chips
- 7 oz. jar marshmallow cream
- 3 cups chopped pecans

Direction

- Bring first 3 ingredients to a boil in a Dutch oven over medium heat, stirring constantly; boil, stirring constantly, 5 minutes.
- Remove from heat; stir in chocolate chips, marshmallow cream and pecans until blended. Pour into a buttered 13X9 pan; let stand at least 2 hours or until firm. Cut into squares.
- Yield: 5 pounds.

48. Chocolate Pecan Toffee Recipe

Serving: 16 | Prep: | Cook: 4mins | Ready in:

Ingredients

- 2 sticks butter
- 1 cup sugar
- 1/4 cup light corn syrup
- 1 cup pecans, finely chopped, divided
- 1 teaspoon vanilla
- 1 1/2 cups milk chocolate chops

Direction

- Coat a 10x15 rimmed baking sheet with non-stick cooking spray
- In a soup pot, combine butter, sugar and corn syrup
- Bring to a boil over medium high heat and boil 3 to 4 minutes, until mixture reaches the hard crack stage, stirring constantly
- Remove mixture from heat and stir 1/2 cup pecans and the vanilla
- Quickly spread over baking sheet
- Sprinkle chocolate chips evenly over mixture and allow to melt; use a knife to spread over toffee, covering completely
- Sprinkle remaining 1/2 cup pecans over melted chocolate then chill at least 1 hour, or until chocolate is firm
- Break into bite-sized pieces and store in an airtight container
- To test for the hard crack stage, drop a bit of the mixture into a glass of cold water, and if it forms a ball that hardens, then it has reached the hard crack stage.

49. Chocolate Truffles

Serving: 0 | Prep: | Cook: | Ready in:

Ingredients

- 3 cups semisweet chocolate chips
- 1 can (14 ounces) sweetened condensed milk
- 1 tablespoon vanilla extract
- Optional coatings: Chocolate sprinkles, Dutch-processed cocoa, espresso powder and cacao nibs

Direction

- In a microwave, melt chocolate chips and milk; stir until smooth. Stir in vanilla. Refrigerate, covered, 2 hours or until firm enough to roll.
- Shape into 1-in. balls. Roll in coatings as desired.
- Nutrition Facts
- 1 truffle: 77 calories, 4g fat (2g saturated fat), 3mg cholesterol, 12mg sodium, 11g carbohydrate (10g sugars, 1g fiber), 1g protein.

50. Chocolate Truffles Recipe

Serving: 8 | Prep: | Cook: | Ready in:

Ingredients

- ½ Cup unsalted butter
- 2 1/3 C confectioner's sugar
- ½ C cocoa
- 1/4 cup heavy or whipping cream 1 1/2 teaspoon vanilla
- Centers: pecan, walnuts, whole almonds or after-dinner mints
- Coatings: coconut, crushed nuts, confectioners sugar

Direction

- Makes about 3 dozen truffles
- Cream butter in large mixer bowl.
- Combine 2 1/2 cups confectioners' sugar and the cocoa; add alternately with cream and vanilla to butter.
- Blend well. Chill until firm. Shape small amount of mixture around desired center; roll into 1 inch balls.
- Drop into desired coating and turn until well covered. Chill until firm.

51. Chocolate Turtle Bars Recipe

Serving: 12 | Prep: | Cook: 20mins | Ready in:

Ingredients

- 1 bag of Rollo chocolate caramel candies, unwrapped
- 2 cups of pecan halves
- 1 cup of chopped pecans
- 1 cup of semi-sweet chocolate chips
- 12 caramel squares, unwrapped
- 1 TB butter

Direction

- Preheat oven to 350 degrees
- Cover an 8x8 inch pan with "release" aluminum foil, leaving extra foil on the sides (to remove candy out of the pan after cooling)
- Pour one cup of pecan halves into the pan, spread out evenly.
- Place the Rollo candies over the pecans.
- Place in oven and cook for 10 minutes at 350 degrees.
- Remove pan from the oven and pour 1 more cup of pecans over the now melted Rollo candies.
- Press the pecans into the Rollos. Set the pan to the side and keep the oven on.
- In a microwave-proof bowl, add the caramels and 1 TB of butter.
- Melt on high for one minute, remove and stir to combine.
- Place back in microwave for 30 seconds.
- Stir well and pour caramel directly over the last layer of pecans.
- Sprinkle the chocolate chips over the caramel evenly.
- Place the pan back into the oven and bake for 5 minutes until the chips look shiny and are beginning to melt.
- Remove pan and spread the chocolate across the surface of the caramel.
- Sprinkle the chopped pecans over the melted chips and using your hands, press them firmly over the warm chocolate.
- Let cool in pan until the chocolate is firm.
- Slice into long bars or into small squares and serve.
- These candies look lovely in clear cellophane bags tied with bows and make a nice food gift. You can freeze these in zip lock bags for months! These are also great for bake sales, potlucks and any family event....

52. Chocolate Butterscotch Pecan Fudge Ala Easy Recipe

Serving: 120 | Prep: | Cook: 5mins | Ready in:

Ingredients

- 1 12-ounce package semi-sweet chocolate chips
- 1 12- ounce package butterscotch chips
- 1 can Eagle Brand milk
- 2 cups chopped pecans (can toast)
- 1/2 stick unsalted butter
- 1 teaspoon vanilla

Direction

- In large bowl, place the chips and Eagle Brand milk.
- Place in microwave to cook.

- Watching closely, stop and stir as needed until melted.
- Remove bowl.
- Stir in butter, stir quickly to mix.
- Add pecans, vanilla.
- Pour into a greased 13x9 dish, or 2-8 inch square dishes.
- Chill until firm, about 2 hours.
- Cut into 1 inch squares, or size of your choice.

53. Chocolate Coconut Truffles Recipe

Serving: 48 | Prep: | Cook: 10mins | Ready in:

Ingredients

- 1 cup (2 sticks) real butter, softened
- 1 pound confectioner's sugar
- 1/2 can sweetened condensed milk
- 1 11-ounce package shredded coconut
- 1 cup chopped pecans (optional)
- 1/2 teaspoon vanilla extract
- 1/4 bar paraffin wax
- 1 16-ounce package semi-sweet chocolate chips
- waxed paper

Direction

- In large mixing bowl, combine softened butter, confectioner's sugar, sweetened condensed milk, coconut, and vanilla, and chopped pecans, if desired. Mix until well blended.
- Refrigerate until firm enough to form balls. (Approximately 1 hour)
- Roll into small balls and place on waxed-paper lined baking sheet.
- Chill once again until firm.
- In double-boiler, melt paraffin wax and chocolate chips until melted and smooth.
- Dip coconut balls into chocolate mixture using toothpicks and place on waxed paper to set.
- May sprinkle additional coconut on top as garnish!
- Refrigerate in plastic container with lid.
- We make several layers with waxed paper to prevent sticking together.
- These also freeze well!

54. Cobblestone Candy Recipe

Serving: 123 | Prep: | Cook: 10mins | Ready in:

Ingredients

- 3-6 ounce packages of semi-sweet chocolate morsel (3 cups)
- 2 cups miniature marshmallows
- 1 cup coarsely chopped nuts; walnut, pecan, peanut, macadamia

Direction

- Melt the semi-sweet morsels in a double boiler.
- Stir until melted and smooth.
- Add marshmallows and nuts.
- Line an 8-inch square pan with aluminum foil.
- Turn chocolate mixture onto the foil-lined pan.
- Let stand until firm.
- Cut into squares.
- Makes 1-2/3 pounds candy.

55. Coconut Pecan Clusters Recipe

Serving: 15 | Prep: | Cook: 5mins | Ready in:

Ingredients

- 1 cup chopped pecans
- 1 cup crisp rice cereal
- 3/4 cup flaked coconut
- 1 package vanilla or white chips, melted

Direction

- Place pecans in a 9 inch pie pan.

- Microwave uncovered on high for 3 to 4 minutes.
- Stir occasionally.
- In a bowl combine the pecans, cereal and coconut
- Add melted chips; mix well.
- Drop by rounded teaspoonfuls onto waxed paper.
- Let stand until set.
- This makes 3 1/2 dozen clusters.

56. Cornflake Candy Recipe

Serving: 4 | Prep: | Cook: 10mins | Ready in:

Ingredients

- 16 ounces milk chocolate, chopped
- 5 cups cornflakes
- 1 cup walnuts, chopped
- 1 cup pecans, chopped

Direction

- Melt milk chocolate in double boiler over low heat. In separate bowl, mix cornflakes and nuts together. Pour melted chocolate over cornflake mixture and stir to coat all ingredients. Drop by the teaspoonful onto a cookie sheet lined with wax paper. Place in the refrigerator to chill and harden. Makes about 48 pieces.

57. Cracker Candy Recipe

Serving: 36 | Prep: | Cook: 5mins | Ready in:

Ingredients

- 1 Container(12-1/2oz) Carmel Topping
- 1 Cup finely chopped pecans(I like cashew as will)
- 3 Dozen round butter-flavored crackers
- 1 package(12oz) semisweet chocolate chips(butterscotch is good too)

Direction

- In a medium saucepan, combine caramel topping and the pecans over medium heat.
- Stirring constantly, bring to a boil and cook 3 to 5 minutes longer or until the mixture thickens.
- Remove from heat and allow to cool 5 minutes.
- Spoon about 1-1/2 teaspoons caramel mixture on top of each cracker.
- Refrigerate 1 hour or until firm.
- In a small saucepan, melt chocolate chips, stirring constantly.
- Remove from heat, dip bottoms of each cracker in chocolate to seal.
- Transfer to waxed paper and refrigerate 1 hour or until chocolate is firm.
- Store in airtight container in refrigerator.
- Makes 3 Dozen Candies

58. Cranberry Candy Recipe

Serving: 50 | Prep: | Cook: 10mins | Ready in:

Ingredients

- 1 can jellied cranberry sauce
- 2 - 3 oz. packages of strawberry jello (or raspberry)
- 1 cup sugar
- 2/3 cup chopped pecans
- sugar

Direction

- Heat jellied cranberry sauce in medium saucepan until melted. Remove from heat and slowly add Jell-O until it is dissolved, then add sugar until it is dissolved. Heat to boiling for 2 minutes. Remove from heat and add pecans, stir well.

- Spray an 8'X8" pan lightly with Pam - don't use a flavored Pam. Pour in cranberry mixture and let it set for 12 hours on the counter in a cool place. Cut in 1" squares and roll in sugar - coating them well.
- Let them ripen for 2 days before eating.

59. Cranberry Coconut Fruit Balls Recipe

Serving: 30 | Prep: | Cook: | Ready in:

Ingredients

- 12 ounces dried apricots
- 1-1/2 cups pecans
- 2 cups fresh cranberries rinsed and drained
- Grated orange peel from 1 orange
- 1/4 cup butter
- 1 pound confectioners' sugar
- 13-1/2 ounces graham cracker crumbs
- 7 ounces coconut flakes

Direction

- Coarsely grind apricots with pecans and cranberries.
- Stir in rind, butter, sugar and crumbs then wrap and chill for 2 hours.
- Shape mixture into 3/4 inch balls.
- Roll balls in coconut.
- Store in refrigerator until ready to serve.

60. Cranberry Fudge Recipe

Serving: 64 | Prep: | Cook: 15mins | Ready in:

Ingredients

- 1¼ cups fresh or frozen cranberries.
- ½ cup light corn syrup
- 2 cups semi-sweet chocolate chips
- ½ cup confectioners (powdered) sugar
- ¼ cup evaporated milk
- 1 teaspoon pure vanilla extract
- ½ cup walnuts or pecans, coarsely chopped (optional)

Direction

- Butter bottom and sides of an 8x8 inch baking pan, or line pan with plastic wrap.
- In a medium sized heavy saucepan over low heat, combine cranberries and corn syrup; bring to a boil, stirring occasionally. Boil about 6 minutes, or until the liquid is reduced to about 3 tablespoons. Remove from heat, immediately add chocolate chips and stir until chocolate is completely melted.
- Add confectioners' sugar, evaporated milk, vanilla, and nuts (optional). Stir vigorously until completely mixed and mixture is thick and glossy.
- Spread into prepared pan. Cover and chill until firm. Cut into 1-inch pieces.
- Makes about 64 one-inch pieces

61. Cranberry Nut Chocolate Bark Recipe

Serving: 12 | Prep: | Cook: 15mins | Ready in:

Ingredients

- 1 cup dried cranberries
- 3/4 cup toasted diced pecans
- 2 2/3 cups chopped semisweet or bittersweet chocolate, melted
- 2 2/3 cups chopped white chocolate, melted

Direction

- Toss the cranberries and pecans together. Set them aside.
- Melt the dark chocolate, and spread it into an 8" x 12" oval on parchment paper.

- Allow the chocolate to set, but not harden completely.
- Melt the white chocolate and mix it with about 3/4 cup of the cranberries and pecans.
- Spread this over the dark chocolate.
- Sprinkle the rest of the nuts and fruit on top, pressing them in gently.
- Allow the candy to cool until hardened, then break it into chunks.

62. Cranberry Nut Fudge Recipe

Serving: 16 | Prep: | Cook: 120mins | Ready in:

Ingredients

- Ingredients:
- 1 tsp. butter
- 1 can (16-oz) milk chocolate frosting
- 1 package (11 ½ -oz) milk chocolate chips
- 1 package (6 -oz) dried cranberries
- ½ cup chopped pecans

Direction

- Line an 8-inch square dish with foil and grease the foil with butter; set aside.
- In a heavy saucepan, combine frosting and chocolate chips. Cook and stir over medium-low heat until chips are melted. Stir in cranberries and nuts. Pour into prepared pan.
- Refrigerate until firm, about 2 hours. Using foil, lift fudge out of pan. Discard foil; cut the fudge into 1-inch squares. Store in the refrigerator. Yields: about 2 pounds.
- Serving size: 1 piece
- Nutritional Values: Calories per serving: 278, Fat: 14g, Cholesterol: 5mg, Sodium: 84mg, Carbohydrate: 38g, Fiber: 2g, Protein: 2g

63. Cream Candy Recipe

Serving: 12 | Prep: | Cook: 10mins | Ready in:

Ingredients

- 2 1/2 cups of sugar
- 1/2 cup of karo
- 1/2 cup of milk
- 6 tablespoons of butter
- vanilla
- 1 large c pecans   (What is a large c?) one full cup, I suppose

Direction

- Her instructions exactly as written:
- Take half butter and toast pecans and salt slightly.
- Boil candy for three minutes-rolling boil-add vanilla; add nuts, beat and beat and beat, then either drop or pour in pan for cutting.
- **
- I toast the chopped pecans in 3 tbsp. of butter
- Combine the sugar, karo, milk, remaining butter in large heavy bottomed sauce pan, bring to rolling boil and time for three minutes. Remove from heat and add vanilla and nuts.
- Beat with a wooden spoon until it becomes pliable and cools down significantly. A real work out for the upper arms.
- Instead of pouring into a 9 x 9. I think it would be better dropped by the spoonful on a sheet of waxed paper to harden.

64. Cream Cheese Fudge Recipe

Serving: 25 | Prep: | Cook: | Ready in:

Ingredients

- 1 - 3 oz. package cream cheese, softened
- 2 cups sifted confectioners sugar

- 1/4 tsp. vanilla flavoring
- a dash of salt
- 1/2 cup chopped pecans
- 2 - 1 oz. squares unsweetened chocolate, melted

Direction

- Cream, cream cheese until smooth.
- Gradually add the sifted confectioners' sugar. Blending well.
- Add melted chocolate and blend well.
- Add vanilla, salt and pecans. Stir well.
- Turn into a well-greased square pan and chill in refrigerator for 30 minutes or until firm.
- Cut into squares.

65. Creme Divinity Kraft Foods Marshmallow Cream Recipe

Serving: 18 | Prep: | Cook: 10mins | Ready in:

Ingredients

- Creme Divinity FROM Kraft foods marshmallow cream
- 1-1/2 cups sugar
- 1/3 cup water
- 1/4 tsp. cream of tartar
- Dash of salt
- 1 jar (7 oz.) JET-PUFFED marshmallow creme
- 1 tsp. vanilla
- 1 cup chopped pecans
- Kraft foods
- Please note, not sure on time, please use a candy thermometer.

Direction

- PLACE sugar, water, cream of tartar and salt in heavy 1-quart saucepan. (Do not stir.) Bring to boil on high heat, without stirring, until candy thermometer registers 248°F.
- BEAT marshmallow crème and vanilla in small bowl with electric mixer on low speed until well blended. Gradually add hot sugar syrup, beating at medium speed until well blended.
- Beat on high speed 5 minutes or until mixture just begins to lose its gloss and hold its shape when dropped from spoon.
- Stir in pecans.
- DROP teaspoonfuls of the marshmallow crème mixture onto sheets of wax paper. Cool completely. Store in airtight container at room temperature.
- Recipe of: Kraft foods

66. Creole Candy Recipe

Serving: 0 | Prep: | Cook: | Ready in:

Ingredients

- One 1 pound box confectioner's sugar
- 1/2 cup (1 stick) butter (do not substitute margarine)
- 1/8 teaspoon salt
- 2 cups pecan halves
- 1/2 cup boiling water
- 1 teaspoon vanilla extract

Direction

- In a large saucepan, combine all the ingredients except the vanilla. Place over medium heat, bring to a boil, then reduce the heat slightly and continue cooking, stirring only enough to prevent scorching, to the soft-ball stage, 238* on a candy thermometer. Remove from the heat, add the vanilla, and stir until the mixture begins to thicken.
- Pour 1 teaspoon of the mixture into each of 36 tiny muffin papers. Allow to cool completely.
- 36 pieces

67. Creole Creamy Pecan Pralines Recipe

Serving: 12 | Prep: | Cook: 15mins | Ready in:

Ingredients

- 1 cup light brown sugar, not packed
- 1 cup sugar
- 1/2 cup evaporated milk
- 3 tbs butter
- 2 tbs light corn syrup
- pinch of salt
- 1 tsp vanilla
- 2 cups pecans, chopped

Direction

- Mix butter, sugars, milk, corn syrup and salt in saucepan and bring to boil stirring with a wooden spoon. Cook to soft ball stage, about 10 minutes. Test by dropping a drop of mixture into cold water. Drop should be soft when picked up with fingers. Remove from heat and add vanilla and nuts. Beat until mixture begins to thicken, about one minute. Drop by tablespoons onto buttered waxed paper. Let cool. ENJOY!
- Note: Put a layer of newspapers under waxed paper. These will spread when dropped.

68. Creole Orange Flavored Pecans Recipe

Serving: 10 | Prep: | Cook: 30mins | Ready in:

Ingredients

- 1 cup sugar
- 1/3 cup fresh orange juice
- 2 tablespoons grated orange peel
- 1-1/2 cups pecan halves

Direction

- Cook sugar, orange juice and orange peel in large saucepan stirring constantly until thread forms when spoon is lifted above pan.
- Add pecan halves and stir until mixture turns to white crystals and nuts cling together.
- Spread and separate on waxed paper covered cookie sheet then cool.

69. Dark Chocolate ButterCrunch Recipe

Serving: 24 | Prep: | Cook: 20mins | Ready in:

Ingredients

- 1 cup (2 sticks, 1/2 pound) butter*
- 1 1/2 cups (12 ounces) sugar
- 3 tablespoons water
- 1 tablespoon light corn syrup
- 2 cups (8 ounces) diced pecans or slivered almonds, toasted
- 1 pound semisweet or bittersweet chocolate, finely chopped (chocolate chips are an easy solution here; you'll need about 2 2/3 cups)
- *If you use unsalted butter, add 1/2 teaspoon salt.

Direction

- In a large, deep saucepan, melt the butter. Stir in the sugar, water and corn syrup, and bring the mixture to a boil. Boil gently, over medium heat, until the mixture reaches hard-crack stage (300°F on an instant-read or candy thermometer), about 20 minutes. The syrup will seem to take a long time to come to the hard-crack stage, but be patient; all of a sudden it will darken, and at that point you need to take its temperature and see if it's ready. (If you don't have a thermometer, test a dollop in ice water; it should immediately harden to a brittleness sufficient that you'll be able to snap it in two, without any bending or softness). Pay attention; too long on the heat,

and the syrup will burn. And what a waste of good butter and sugar that would be!
- While the sugar mixture is gently bubbling, spread half of the nuts, in a fairly closely packed, even single layer, on a lightly greased baking sheet. Top with half the chocolate. When the syrup is ready, pour it quickly and evenly over the nuts and chocolate. Immediately top with the remaining chocolate, then the remaining nuts. Wait several minutes, then gently, using the back of a spatula, press down on the chocolate-nut layer to spread the chocolate around evenly.
- While the candy is still slightly warm, use a spatula to loosen it from the baking sheet. When cool, break it into uneven chunks.
- Yield: about 24 big bite-sized pieces, if you want to be scientific about it.

70. Dark Chocolate Cococans Recipe

Serving: 30 | Prep: | Cook: 10mins | Ready in:

Ingredients

- 1 14 ounce bag of sweetened shredded coconut
- 1 bag of dark chocolate chips-you can use semi-sweet
- 6 ounces of sweetened condensed milk
- 1/2 tsp vanilla extract
- 1/2 tsp almond extract
- 2 cups of powdered sugar
- 1 pound of large pecan halves
- 1/4 cup of honey
- 1/4 tsp. salt
- (butter for your hands!)

Direction

- Mix the condensed milk with the sugar
- Add extracts and salt and mix well.
- Press this mixture evenly into a 13x9 pan covered in Release aluminum foil with extra foil on sides for easy removal.
- Place in the freezer for one hour.
- Remove the pan from the freezer and remove the candy from the pan using the foil.
- Cut into small 2 inch squares
- Using buttered hands, roll the candy into small log-shaped pieces, rounding off the edges slightly.
- Dip only the bottom of one pecan half lightly into the honey and press on top of each coconut log or piece. (Honey is the glue!)
- Place all of the candy on wax paper or a silicon mat (or use the foil!)
- Melt the dark chocolate in a glass bowl or large glass measuring cup.
- Using 2 forks, quickly dip each candy and pecan into the chocolate and allow excess to drip off.
- Place dipped candy back on foil or waxed paper to dry and set.

71. Date Drops Recipe

Serving: 6 | Prep: | Cook: 5mins | Ready in:

Ingredients

- 2 eggs beaten
- 1/3 cup butter
- 1/2 cup black dates finely cut
- 1-1/2 cups crisp rice cereal
- 1/2 cup pecans chopped
- 1 teaspoon vanilla

Direction

- Combine eggs, butter and dates. Cook over low heat stirring constantly. Boil for 2 minutes. Remove from heat and add cereal, nuts and vanilla. Cool then shape into balls.

72. Delicious Homemade Creme Filled Chocolate Candy Recipe

Serving: 24 | Prep: | Cook: 5mins | Ready in:

Ingredients

- Centers:
- 1 cup of sweetened condensed milk
- 1/4 lb softened margarine
- 2 1/2 lbs powdered sugar
- 1 tsp vanilla (or any extract you'd like! mint or maple are great inside chocolates!)
- 1/2 cup of ground up pecan or walnut halves- optional

Direction

- Blend ingredients, then shape into 1" balls and chill for a few hours or overnight.
- Using a toothpick, dip each ball into the chocolate (recipe below) and cool on waxed paper or tin foil.
- (Cover the toothpick hole with a little teensy bit more of the chocolate, using the toothpick)
- Chocolate:
- 12 oz. of semi-sweet bits
- 6 oz. unsweetened chocolate
- Melt in microwave or in a double boiler to dip the centers (above) in! Keep the chocolate warm while dipping centers.

73. Divine Divinity Recipe

Serving: 36 | Prep: | Cook: 25mins | Ready in:

Ingredients

- 2 1/2 cups sugar
- 2/3 cup light corn syrup
- 1/2 cup water
- 2 large egg whites
- 1 1/2 teaspoons vanilla
- 2/3 cup coarsely chopped pecans or walnuts or chopped red or green candied cherries (optional)

Direction

- Step 1:
- Line a baking sheet with waxed paper. In a large heavy saucepan, combine the sugar, corn syrup, and water. Bring to a boil over moderately high heat, stirring constantly with a wooden spoon to dissolve sugar. (Avoid splashing mixture onto side of the pan.) Boil for 3 minutes. If using a candy thermometer, carefully clip to side of pan, making sure the bulb is immersed but not touching the bottom of the pan.
- Step 2:
- Cook over moderate heat, without stirring, to 260 on candy thermometer, hard-ball stage (15 to 18 minutes). (Or, use this cold water test. Using a spoon, drop a small amount of hot mixture into very cold, not icy, water. Dip your fingers into the water and form the mixture into a ball. Remove the ball from the water; it should not flatten but can be deformed by pressure.)
- Step 3:
- Remove pan from heat; remove the thermometer from saucepan. In a large bowl, with very clean beaters and an electric mixer on medium to high, beat the egg whites until stiff peaks form. Slowly pour hot syrup mixture in a fine stream over egg whites, beating with electric mixer on high for 3 minutes and scraping the side of the bowl occasionally.
- Step 4:
- Add the vanilla. Continue beating with the electric mixer on high just until candy starts to lose its gloss and holds soft peaks (5 to 6 minutes), scraping the side of the bowl occasionally. Stir in nuts (if using).
- Step 5:
- Working quickly, drop by teaspoonfuls onto waxed paper. If the divinity becomes too stiff, beat in very hot water, a few drops at a time,

until it is a softer consistency. Cool completely. To store, cover tightly.
- Notes:
- Choose a dry day. Because sugar absorbs moisture from the air, divinity may never set up if you try to make it on a humid day.
- Start with room temperature egg whites. They heat up to a greater volume than cold egg whites
- Use a heavy-duty, freestanding electric mixer. Beating divinity puts a strain on a mixer's motor. Portable mixers and lightweight, freestanding mixers may not have heavy enough motors.
- Follow the recipe directions carefully. Timing is important. Adding the hot syrup too quickly or not beating the candy mixture long enough can cause divinity to fail. Overbeating the divinity will cause it to set up before you can drop it into individual pieces.
- ....

74. Double Nut English Toffee Recipe

Serving: 28 | Prep: | Cook: 15mins | Ready in:

Ingredients

- 1 1/2 teaspoons plus 2 - cups butter softened and divided
- 2- cups granulated sugar
- 1- cup chopped almonds
- 1- package (12 ounces) semi-sweet chocolate chips...divided.....
- 2- cups pecans or you can use walnuts.... divided ....(i like the pecans),

Direction

- Butter a 15 inch x 10 inch x 1 inch pan with 1 1/2 teaspoons butter set aside
- In a heavy saucepan, combine sugar and remaining butter

- Cook and stir over medium heat until a candy thermometer reads 290 degrees (soft crack stage)
- Remove from heat stir in almonds
- Immediately pour into prepared pan
- Sprinkle with 1 cup of the chocolate chips let stand until the chips become glossy, spread evenly over the top
- Sprinkle with 1 cup pecans
- Cover and refrigerate until set about 1 hour
- In microwave melt remaining chips
- Stir until smooth
- Spread over toffee and sprinkle with remaining pecans. Cover and refrigerate again for 30 minutes
- Then break into 2 inch pieces
- Store in an airtight container
- Yields 3 1/2 pounds candy

75. Double Nut English Toffee Recipe Recipe

Serving: 30 | Prep: | Cook: | Ready in:

Ingredients

- • 2 - cups butter softened and divided
- • 2 cups sugar
- • 1- package (12 ounces) semi-sweet chocolate chips...... (I needed another 12 ounces)
- • 2- cups pecans or you can use walnuts.... divided .... (I liked the pecans), I had about 1/4 cup left over.
- • Wooden spoon (I prefer bamboo spoons)
- Here is Tinks link if you want to comment on this recipe she posted.
- Double Nut English Toffee

Direction

- Butter a 15 inch x 10 inch x 1 inch pan with 1 1/2 teaspoons butter set aside. I took it I was to spread out the butter using my fingers per the picture, or maybe just getting the thinnest layer and only using 1/2 teaspoon..... Once

made, the bottom seemed greasy; I would like to try just spraying canola oil on the bottom, a very light coat and spreading it out very thin. There is so much butter in the recipe I wonder if it would really stick inside the pan?
- In a heavy saucepan, combine sugar and remaining butter
- Cook and stir over medium heat until a candy thermometer reads 290 degrees (soft crack stage). I used my 2 quart copper bottom and after 30 minutes on medium and medium high my candy thermometer would not go past 225. At 30 minutes it had been bubbling and started to change consistency, it began balling up on the wooden spoon. I decided that was it, and poured it on the buttered sheet. It spread out very nice.
- Sprinkle with 1 cup (I think another 6-8 ounces) of the chocolate chips, let stand until the chips become glossy........spread evenly over the top. I think it would have been better to nuke the chips and soften them a little; about 30-45 seconds so they would melt better on the mixture and spread out easier and more even. If you look closely there are areas where the chips didn't fill the whole mix. They did get glossy per the original recipe. Add nuts
- I placed the whole tray in the refrigerator for 1 hour to set up.
- Remove from refrigerator.
- It does make over 3 lbs. and is quite thick. It has incredible flavor, but then how could 2 lbs. of real butter and 2 cups of sugar not taste good. This was totally low cal and non-fatting good stuff.
- Break into 2 inch pieces or whatever and store in an airtight container
- Yields 3 1/2 pounds candy.

76. Dr Pepper Pralines Recipe

Serving: 6 | Prep: | Cook: 20mins | Ready in:

Ingredients

- 1 cup white sugar
- 1 cup dark brown sugar
- 1 cup Dr. pepper
- 4 large marshmallows
- 3 cups pecan halves

Direction

- In heavy saucepan mix together sugars and Dr Pepper.
- Cook over low heat stirring constantly until all sugar is dissolved then cook stirring occasionally until softball stage reached.
- Remove from heat and add marshmallows and nutmeats together.
- Beat hard for 2 minutes.
- Drop on waxed paper in small balls 1 tablespoon at a time.
- They should flatten out around the edges leaving mound of nutmeats in center.

77. Dressed Up Chocolate Bark Recipe

Serving: 12 | Prep: | Cook: 10mins | Ready in:

Ingredients

- chocolate (milk or semi-sweet)
- Classic Toppings: dried fruits such as apricots, raisins, candied orange peel, cranberries, and cherries. toasted nuts including hazelnuts, pecans, almonds, and pistachios.
- Contemporary Toppings: caramelized cocoa nibs (see recipe), cereal, candied ginger, and dried fruits such as pineapple, blueberries, and strawberries. toasted pumpkin seeds and pine nuts.

Direction

- Line a chilled baking sheet with parchment paper. Pour warm (not hot), melted chocolate into the prepared pan.

- Spread the chocolate evenly to about 1/8 inch thick using a small offset spatula. Sprinkle toppings on the chocolate and place in the freezer to set, approximately 20 minutes.
- For even-sized pieces, cut up bark before it sets completely. If you like a more rustic look, allow the bark to harden completely before breaking it up into pieces. Store in a cool, dry place.

78. Easy Apricot Balls Recipe

Serving: 1 | Prep: | Cook: | Ready in:

Ingredients

- 8 ounces dried apricots, finely chopped
- 1 cup sweetened flaked coconut
- 1/2 cup chopped walnuts
- 2 tab fresh squeesed orange juice
- 1/4 cup sweetened condensed milk
- more flaked coconut or finely chopped pecans for rolling
- Optional (dip cold balls in melted chocolate and roll in coconut or chopped nuts)

Direction

- Process chopped apricots, walnuts and coconut in a food processor until thoroughly combined. Add OJ and sweetened condensed milk; process until combined. Pour mixture into a dish; refrigerate until firm, about 30 to 45 minutes. Place waxed paper on a baking sheet; set aside. Place additional coconut or finely chopped pecans in a shallow bowl. Shape apricot mixture into balls about 1-inch in diameter. Roll in coconut or pecans; place on waxed paper. Refrigerate until firm. Store in an airtight container in the refrigerator. Makes about 24 balls.

79. Easy Chocolate Fudge Recipe

Serving: 1 | Prep: | Cook: 10mins | Ready in:

Ingredients

- 1 lb powdered sugar, sifted
- ½ cup cocoa powder, sifted
- 1 stick (1/2 cup) butter, cubed into small chunks
- ¼ cup chocolate milk, plain milk works fine, too (I used skim, but anything will work)
- 1 tablespoon vanilla
- ½ cup chopped pecans, optional

Direction

- First, set out your ingredients: sifted powdered sugar and cocoa, cubed butter, chocolate milk (regular is fine, too!), and vanilla.
- You can add pecans, or any nut meats, if you so desire.
- Place all of your ingredients in a microwavable bowl, minus the vanilla and optional nut meats.
- Microwave for 90 seconds.
- During this 90 seconds, line a small pan (I used a 6 x 8) with saran wrap.
- Remove from the microwave and whisk until smooth.
- Then stir in vanilla and optional nuts.
- Pour into the saran wrapped pan, cover and place in the refrigerator until hardened. Slice, serve, and go nuts! Or…don't go nuts…
- This easy chocolate fudge is ultra-thick, smooth, creamy, and extra chocolaty.

80. Easy Chocolate Macaroons Recipe

Serving: 30 | Prep: | Cook: 30mins | Ready in:

Ingredients

- 2 squares BAKER'S unsweetened chocolate
- 1 can (300 mL) sweetened condensed milk
- 2 squares BAKER'S white chocolate, chopped
- 2 cups flaked coconut
- 1 cup chopped pecans

Direction

- Preheat oven to 350°F.
- Microwave unsweetened chocolate and milk in large microwaveable bowl on HIGH 2 min. or until chocolate is almost melted.
- Stir until chocolate is completely melted.
- Stir in remaining ingredients.
- Drop by heaping teaspoonfuls, 2 inches apart, onto greased baking sheets.
- Bake 10 to 12 min. or until tops are set.
- Immediately remove from baking sheets to wire racks. Cool completely.

81. Easy Delicious Nutty Marshmallow Log Recipe

Serving: 100 | Prep: | Cook: 20mins | Ready in:

Ingredients

- 2 cups chopped pecans
- About 1-1/4 cups powdered sugar, divided
- 1 (16 ounce) package marshmallows
- 3-4 tablespoons peanut butter

Direction

- Combine pecans and 1 cup powdered sugar
- Sprinkle the above mixture evenly over a large sheet of waxed paper
- Place marshmallows in top of double boiler, bring water to boil
- Reduce heat to low; cook until marshmallows melt
- Stir in peanut butter
- Pour marshmallow mixture over powdered sugar pecan mixture
- Mix with hands, until pecans and sugar are blended into marshmallow mixture and mixture resembles soft dough
- Shape into 2 rolls, 1 inch in diameter
- Let stand about 45 minutes
- Roll candy in remaining powdered sugar
- Let stand at least 30 minutes
- Cut into 1/4 inch slices
- Store in a covered container, separating layers with waxed paper

82. Easy Microwave Pralines Recipe

Serving: 24 | Prep: | Cook: 8mins | Ready in:

Ingredients

- 1 1/2 cups brown sugar
- 2/3 cup heavy cream
- 2 tablespoons butter
- 1 cup pecan halves

Direction

- In a large, microwave safe bowl, combine sugar, cream, butter, pecans.
- Microwave 8 minutes on high, stirring once.
- Let rest 1 minute
- Then stir 3 minutes more.
- Drop by teaspoonfuls on buttered waxed paper (If mixture is runny, allow to cool 30 seconds more and try again.)

83. Easy Peanut Butter Chocolate Fudge Recipe

Serving: 0 | Prep: | Cook: 20mins | Ready in:

Ingredients

- 1 (12 ounce) package peanut butter flavored chips
- 1/4 cup butter

- 1 (14 ounce) can sweetened condensed milk
- 1/2 cup chopped pecans (optional)
- 1 (6 ounce) package semi-sweet chocolate chips (1 cup)

Direction

- 1. Line an 8 inch square pan with wax paper.
- 2. In a microwavable safe bowl put the peanut butter chips, 1 cup of the condensed milk and 2 tablespoons butter and put in microwave for about 1 minute (time may vary depending on your microwave)
- 3. When done stir all the ingredients together and spread mixture into pan.
- 4. Then place the pan in the fridge to chill whilst you make the chocolate mixture for the top.
- 5. In another bowl place the chocolate chips the remaining condensed milk and 2 tablespoons of butter and place in microwave for the same amount of time.
- 6. When done spread the mixture on top of the peanut butter evenly.
- 7. Then place back in the fridge to chill for about 2 hours.
- 8. Then remove and turn out fudge onto chopping board remove the wax paper and cut.

84. Easy Peanut Butter Fudge

Serving: 8 | Prep: | Cook: 30mins | Ready in:

Ingredients

- 2 teaspoons butter, softened
- 2 cups sugar
- 1/2 cup whole milk
- 1-1/3 cups peanut butter
- 1 jar (7 ounces) marshmallow creme

Direction

- Line an 8-in. square pan with foil; grease with butter.
- In a heavy saucepan, combine sugar and milk; bring to a boil over medium heat, stirring constantly. Boil 3 minutes, stirring constantly. Remove from heat.
- Stir in peanut butter and marshmallow creme until blended. Immediately spread into prepared pan; cool slightly.
- Refrigerate until firm. Using foil, lift fudge out of pan. Remove foil; cut into squares. Store between layers of waxed paper in an airtight container.
- Tips:
- Drizzle individual fudge squares with melted chocolate to add some easy holiday glam.
- We tasted six popular kinds of chunky peanut butter. Here's the brand we like best.
- Nutrition Facts
- 1 piece: 67 calories, 3g fat (1g saturated fat), 0 cholesterol, 28mg sodium, 10g carbohydrate (9g sugars, 0 fiber), 1g protein.

85. Easy Toffee Recipe

Serving: 20 | Prep: | Cook: 7mins | Ready in:

Ingredients

- 3/4 cup brown sugar (packed)
- 1/2 cup butter
- 1 cup chopped walnuts (or pecans)
- 1/2 cup semi sweet chocolate chips

Direction

- Grease a 9 x 9-inch cake pan.
- Spread the chopped walnuts evenly in the bottom of the pan.
- Over high heat, melt together sugar and butter in medium size saucepan until boiling.
- Lower heat to medium.
- Boil over medium heat for 7 minutes.
- Pour into pan.
- Sprinkle chocolate chips over hot mixture.

- Place a cookie sheet over the pan to retain the heat and melt the chocolate chips.
- Cut into large squares while hot, then refrigerate until hard.
- Break into pieces.

86. Elegant Marshmallows Recipe

Serving: 20 | Prep: | Cook: 10mins | Ready in:

Ingredients

- 1 bag of fresh large marshmallows
- 3 cups of your choice of chocolate for dipping
- *Toppings:
- Finely chopped pecans, walnuts, macadamia nuts or peanuts
- toasted and finely chopped almonds
- Dark or milk chocolate sprinkles
- graham cracker crumbs
- toasted coconut
- Colored sugar crystals
- Toffee bits, finly chopped

Direction

- Prepare your work area first by laying down either sheets of wax paper or aluminum foil to catch any drips. Have some paper-lined trays and some wire racks ready.
- You'll need two forks.
- Put your toppings into cereal or soup-sized bowls. You will need room to roll the chocolate-dipped marshmallows into your toppings.
- Put your chocolate into the microwave for one minute.
- Remove and stir until melted.
- If the chocolate hasn't melted, cook for 30 more seconds and stir.
- Drop one marshmallow directly into the chocolate and dip it quickly, rolling it around until completely covered.
- Let the excess chocolate drip off and place on wire rack.
- If at any time, your chocolate gets too firm to roll, place it back in the microwave for about 10 seconds and stir.
- If you want to dip the marshmallow into one of your toppings, as soon as it is covered in chocolate, with the two forks, drop the marshmallow directly into the topping and roll until covered in nuts, crumbs or sprinkles and place on tray to dry.
- That's all there is to it!
- - I enjoy using the Lindt chocolate candy bars that come out during the holidays as the chocolate is fantastic and very creamy. You have to make sure that you don't over heat it in the microwave or it can burn. Better chocolate makes for a better dipped marshmallow!
- I place several varieties of marshmallows in clear cellophane bags and give them out to as gifts for the holidays. These can be shipped in candy boxes well during the cooler months.
- -

87. Elegant Martha Washington Candy Recipe

Serving: 0 | Prep: | Cook: 60mins | Ready in:

Ingredients

- For nougat::
- 4 cups powdered sugar
- 1/2 cup melted butter
- 2 cups sweetened flaked coconut
- 3 cups chopped pecans
- 1 (14 ounce) can sweetened condensed milk
- Mix all ingredients in a LARGE bowl....dishpan size if you have it.
- I used the same bowl that I mix my Thanksgiving dressing up in.
- Form in one inch balls and place on a baking sheet that's been lined with waxed paper or a baking mat.

Direction

- For chocolate coating:
- 16 ounces semi-sweet chocolate morsels
- 1 1/2 cakes paraffin wax
- Melt chocolate and paraffin wax in a double boiler stirring frequently.
- When melted, use toothpicks to dip nougat balls in wax. Place on waxed paper to dry.
- You'll have coating left over after all the nougat balls are dipped. If you have pretzels on hand, you can give them a chocolate coating, too. Paraffin wax helps the chocolate stay nice and liquid which makes coating easier. After dipping, it makes the chocolate harden faster and keeps it from melting in your hands.

88. English Toffee Recipe

Serving: 6 | Prep: | Cook: 1hours | Ready in:

Ingredients

- 2 cup sugar
- 4 sticks butter
- 2 half-pound bars of Hershey's Symphony milk chocolate
- 1 cup chopped pecans (optional)

Direction

- Cover a large cookie with foil, grease foil.
- Sprinkle chopped pecans on pan if desired.
- Break up chocolate into a glass bowl, ready to melt quickly in the microwave.
- Melt butter in a Dutch oven. Do NOT use teflon!
- Add the sugar and stir constantly with a wooden spoon.
- The butter and sugar will slowly combine, separate, and combine again.
- Once combined for good and a toffee color (around 330 degrees on a candy thermometer), pour into cookie sheet and spread it out.
- Microwave the chocolate for 2 minutes, or melt as desired.
- Once ready, spread over the top of the toffee.
- Let cool in refrigerator.
- Once cool, break into pieces to serve.

89. Extravagant Old Fashioned Fudge Dated 1942 Recipe

Serving: 12 | Prep: | Cook: 20mins | Ready in:

Ingredients

- 2 cups granulated sugar
- 1 cup milk
- 1/2-teaspoon salt
- 2 squares unsweetened chocolate
- 2 tablespoons white corn syrup
- 2 tablespoons butter
- 1/2 teaspoon vanilla extract
- 1/2 cup chopped pecans

Direction

- In saucepan combine sugar, milk, salt, chocolate and corn syrup.
- Stir over low heat until sugar dissolves.
- Cook gently stirring occasionally until a mixture dropped into cold water forms soft ball.
- Remove from heat and drop in butter but do not stir then cool without stirring.
- Add vanilla then with spoon beat until candy loses gloss then add nuts.
- Turn into greased loaf pan then cool and cut into squares.

90. Fudge Recipe

Serving: 1 | Prep: | Cook: 25mins | Ready in:

Ingredients

- 2 cups sugar
- 1 cup whipping cream
- 3 Tbsp. butter
- 1-1/2 squares unsweetened chocolate
- Note: I have used unsweetened, milk and white chocolate for this recipe.
- 2 Tbsp. white Karo syrup
- 1-1/2 tsp. vanilla
- 1 cup chopped pecans (optional)
- Note: Instead of adding pecans I like to add miniature marshmallows!!! I have even added a combination of maraschino cherries(well drained and quarted) plus marshmallows.

Direction

- Grease sides and bottom of 3 qt. heavy saucepan.
- Add sugar, cream, butter, chocolate and Karo syrup.
- Stir, being careful not to get sugar mixture on greased sides of pan. Bring to a boil over medium heat and cook to 230-238 degrees F on candy thermometer, stirring occasionally to keep candy from sticking.
- Remove from heat, pour candy immediately into mixing bowl.
- Add vanilla and beat with mixer until candy loses the gloss.
- Add pecans (optional) and pour into greased an 8 x 8 inch pan.
- Cut when cool.

91. Graham Break Aways Recipe

Serving: 24 | Prep: | Cook: 25mins | Ready in:

Ingredients

- 12 honey graham crackers broken in half (24 pieces)
- 1/2 c. butter
- 3/4 c. packed brown sugar
- 1 c. semi-sweet chocolate chips
- 1/2 c. finely chopped pecans or other nuts (optional)

Direction

- Preheat oven to 350. Arrange graham crackers in a single layer on a cookie sheet.
- In a medium sauce pan, bring butter and sugar to a boil over medium heat, cook 2 minutes.
- Pour over grahams and spread quickly to cover all the crackers.
- Bake 6-8 minutes or until sugar mixture is slightly browned and bubbly.
- Remove and sprinkle with chocolate chips
- Bake another 1-2 minutes until chocolate is melted.
- Remove from oven and spread chocolate, add nuts if desired.
- Cool completely and break into squares.
- Enjoy!

92. Graham Cracker Brittle Recipe

Serving: 10 | Prep: | Cook: 8mins | Ready in:

Ingredients

- Pre Heat Oven 350
- 10 graham crackers
- 2 Sticks butter
- 1/2 cup chopped nuts, I use pecans
- 1 tsp vanilla
- 1/2 cup sugar

Direction

- Lay graham crackers to one side of cookie sheet.
- In sauce pan melt butter till bubbling.
- Add sugar and stir.
- Stirring add nuts and cook 3 minutes.
- Add Vanilla stirring for another 3 minutes.
- Pour evenly over graham crackers.
- Bake 8-10 minutes.
- Let cool and break into pieces.

- Cool and enjoy!

93. Graham Cracker Nut Brittle Recipe

Serving: 1012 | Prep: | Cook: 10mins | Ready in:

Ingredients

- 1 box graham crackers
- 1 Cup chopped pecans
- 3/4 Cup butter
- 1/2 Cup margarine
- 1/2 Cup granulated sugar
- 1 teaspoon vanilla

Direction

- Preheat oven to 350 degrees F. Line cookie sheet with parchment paper for easy clean-up.
- Layer a 17 X 11 inch cookie sheet with graham cracker squares. Sprinkle nuts over the graham crackers. Combine butter, margarine & sugar in a pot and cook until butter is melted and blended well. Boil 2 minutes. Pour over the crackers and nuts. Bake in preheated oven for 10 minutes. Remove and cool for 5 minutes. Transfer to wax paper to cool or this will stick.

94. Graham Cracker Snacks Recipe

Serving: 12 | Prep: | Cook: 25mins | Ready in:

Ingredients

- 2 cups graham cracker crumbs, crushed
- 1 1/2 pecans, chopped
- 1 can Eagle Brand sweetened condensed milk

Direction

- Mix all ingredients together.
- Place in greased 8x8 baking dish.
- Bake at 325 degrees for 25 minutes.

95. Heirloom Cream Candy Recipe

Serving: 18 | Prep: | Cook: 10mins | Ready in:

Ingredients

- 2 1/2 cups of sugar
- 1/2 cup of Karo syrup
- 1/2 cup of milk
- 3/4 stick of butter
- vanilla
- 1 large c pecans

Direction

- Take half butter and toast pecan & salt slightly.
- Boil candy for 3 minutes-rolling boil-add vanilla & add nuts, beat and beat, then either drop or pour in pan for cutting.

96. Holiday Candy Fudge Bars Recipe

Serving: 3 | Prep: | Cook: 25mins | Ready in:

Ingredients

- 2 cups uncooked quick-cooking oats
- 1 1/2 cups all-purpose flour
- 1 cup chopped pecans
- 1 cup firmly packed light brown sugar
- 1 teaspoon baking soda
- 1/4 teaspoon salt
- 1 cup butter/margarine, melted
- 1 1/2 cups red and green M&M's, divided
- 1 (14-ounce) can sweetened condensed milk

Direction

- Combine first 6 ingredients, stirring well. Add butter, and stir or beat at low speed with an electric mixer until mixture is crumbly. Reserve 1 1/2 cups crumb mixture; press remaining crumb mixture into a lightly greased 13x9 pan. Bake at 375 for 10 minutes. Cool on a wire rack. Reduce oven temperature to 350.
- Place 1 cup chocolate pieces in a microwave-safe bowl, microwave at High 1 to 1 1/2 minutes, stirring after 30 seconds. Press chocolate pieces with the back of a spoon to mash them (the candies will almost be melted with pieces of color coating still visible). Stir in condensed milk. Spread evenly over crust in pan, leaving 1/2inch border on all sides.
- Combine reserved 1 1/2 cups crumb mixture and remaining 1/2 cup of M&M's; sprinkle evenly over chocolate mixture, and press lightly.
- Bake at 350 for 25 to 28 minutes or until golden; cool in pan on wire rack. Cut into bars.

97. Homemade Cinnamon Praline Pecans Recipe

Serving: 20 | Prep: | Cook: 30mins | Ready in:

Ingredients

- 2 lbs pecan or walnut halves
- 2 egg whites
- 2 tsp water
- 1 cup sugar
- 1 tsp cinnamon
- a dash of salt
- 1/2 tsp cocoa-or more
- cayenne pepper to taste

Direction

- Preheat oven to 325.
- Beat egg whites and water together.
- Stir in pecans and toss quickly.
- In the meantime, have mixed the sugar, cinnamon, salt and cocoa. Pour over the pecans and toss quickly.
- Pour pecans into a greased baking sheet.
- Bake about 30 minutes, stirring every ten minutes.
- Using a spatula, loosen the pecans from the sheet immediately. Cool.
- Can be stored in an airtight container for up to two weeks.
- You can use any nuts you like, really. I love cashews done this way, too.

98. Honey Macadamia Nut Fudge Recipe

Serving: 36 | Prep: | Cook: 30mins | Ready in:

Ingredients

- 1-1/2 cups granulated sugar
- 1 cup packed brown sugar
- 1/3 cup half-and-half or light cream
- 1/3 cup milk
- 2 tablespoons honey
- 2 tablespoons butter
- 1 teaspoon vanilla
- 1/2 cup coarsely chopped macadamia nuts, hazelnuts (filberts), or pecans
- Chopped nuts or chopped dried pineapple or papaya (optional)

Direction

- 1. Line a 9x5x3-inch loaf pan with foil, extending foil over edges of the pan. Butter the foil; set pan aside.
- 2. Butter the sides of a heavy 2-quart saucepan. In the saucepan, combine granulated sugar, brown sugar, half-and-half or light cream, milk, and honey. Cook and stir over medium-high heat until mixture boils and sugars dissolve (about 8 minutes). Clip a candy thermometer to side of pan. Reduce heat to medium-low; continue to boil at a moderate

steady rate, stirring frequently, until thermometer registers 234 degrees F, soft-ball stage (15 to 20 minutes). Adjust heat as necessary to maintain a steady boil.
- 3. Remove pan from heat. Add butter and vanilla, but do not stir. Cool, without stirring, to 110 degrees F (50 to 60 minutes).
- 4. Remove thermometer from pan. Beat mixture vigorously with a clean wooden spoon until fudge just begins to thicken; stir in the 1/2 cup nuts. Continue beating until fudge just starts to lose its gloss (about 10 minutes total).
- 5. Immediately spread fudge evenly in prepared pan. Score into 1-1/4-inch squares while warm, and if desired, sprinkle with additional nuts or dried fruit. When fudge is firm, use foil to lift it out of the pan. Cut fudge into squares. Makes 1-1/4 pounds (about 36 pieces).
- To store: Store in an airtight container at room temperature for up to 1 week

melted. Be careful not to let milk or marshmallows burn.
- Remove from heat.
- Add chips, 1 bag at a time, stirring briefly between each back.
- Stir slowly, but firmly, until chocolate is completely melted.
- Add nuts and vanilla and stir well, to combine.
- Pour(dump :) mixture into thoroughly buttered and parchment(wax) papered 9X13 glass baking dish or, for thinner fudge, you can use an 11X14 high sided baking sheet, or 2 8X8 or 9X9 square cake or glass pans.
- Cool at least a few hours, then turn over onto clean surface and cut into squares.*
- *If you're worried about the fudge coming out of the pan, then use the parchment or wax paper, and leave the short sides up over the top of the fudge so you can "lift" it out of the pan. OR, carefully cut one corner, grab hold of the paper, there, and it should pop right out.

99. I Forgot To Make The Fudge Recipe

Serving: 48 | Prep: | Cook: 15mins | Ready in:

Ingredients

- 6 cups (1 package) miniature marshmallows
- 2 14oz cans sweetened condensed milk
- 1/2t salt
- 2 12oz packages semi sweet chocolate chips
- 1 12oz package milk chocolate chips
- 1/2 cup toasted nuts(walnuts, pecans, etc)- optional
- 2t vanilla

Direction

- Heat milk, marshmallows and salt in large saucepan over medium low heat. Cook, stirring frequently, until marshmallows are

100. Inside Out Caramel Apples Recipe

Serving: 24 | Prep: | Cook: 25mins | Ready in:

Ingredients

- 3 large apples
- 1 lemon
- 2 cups brown sugar
- 1/2 cup heavy cream
- 2 tbsp butter
- 2 tbsp corn syrup
- 1 tsp vanilla extract
- 1/4 cup chopped pecans or walnuts
- melted chocolate or almond bark

Direction

- Cut your apples in half. Using a melon baller, scoop out the insides, leaving a 1/2 to 1/4 inch thickness.

- Squeeze the juice from the lemon onto the apples and allow to set. It will keep them from browning right away.
- In a sauce pan over high heat, add the brown sugar, butter, heavy cream and corn syrup. Stir until the brown sugar has dissolved. Allow to boil, stirring occasionally, until it reaches 230 degrees, about 7-10 minutes. Remove from heat and add the vanilla, stir continually until it stops bubbling. Allow to cool for about 10-15 minutes.
- Wipe your apples down with a paper towel, removing as much lemon juice as possible. Caramel won't stick to a wet apple.
- Pour the caramel into the apples leaving a small space at the top.
- Sprinkle with pecans.
- Refrigerate until the caramel has set.
- Cut into slices and drizzle melted chocolate over each slice.

101. Louisiana Pralines Recipe

Serving: 24 | Prep: | Cook: | Ready in:

Ingredients

- 2 cups powdered sugar
- 1 cup maple syrup
- 1/2 cup cream
- 2 cups pecan halves

Direction

- Combine Powdered Sugar and cream. Add maple syrup and boil to soft ball-stage (236°F). Then beat until mixture begins to sugar. Add nuts and drop on greased waxed paper into two-inch patties. Wrap individually in plastic wrap. Makes about twenty-four.

102. Macadamia Cashew Crunch Recipe

Serving: 6 | Prep: | Cook: 20mins | Ready in:

Ingredients

- 2 cups bittersweet or semi-sweet chocolate (The orig. recipe used milk chocolate chips.)
- 1 cup chopped salted macadamia nuts
- 1 cup chopped salted cashews
- 1/2 cup sugar
- 1/2 stick softened butter - do not substitute margarine
- 2 TB corn syrup
- *Options:
- This can be made with walnuts, pecans or even peanuts. You can use nuts that are not salted in this recipe.

Direction

- Line a 9 inch pan with "release" aluminum, making sure that the foil goes over the edge of the pan so that you can pick the candy out of the pan with ease. You can butter regular foil and use that instead.
- Sprinkle the bottom of the pan with the chocolate chips.
- Place your butter, sugar, corn syrup and nuts in a large and heavy skillet and cook over low heat.
- Stir constantly until the butter melts and the sugar dissolves. (10-12 minutes on my stovetop)
- Increase the heat to medium and stir constantly until the candy turns into a light golden brown color.
- Watch the candy carefully and stir when the candy starts to stick together. It will get harder to stir at this point.
- Pour the mixture over the chocolate in the pan.
- Spread the candy evenly over the chips. Do not mash the chips and allow them to melt on their own.
- Let this all cool for at least one hour and then refrigerate until firm.

- Remove from pan, peel off the foil and break into pieces or cut into squares.
- ***** I have to add this. I over-cooked this once because I could not get a golden "brown" color out of the sugar mass. It came out like a thick brittle after I refrigerated it and tried to cut it. So watch your candy while it cooks. It was still good but be careful!

103. Maple Pecan Fudge Recipe

Serving: 64 | Prep: | Cook: 80mins | Ready in:

Ingredients

- 4 TBSP. unsalted butter, softened
- 3/4 c. pure maple syrup
- 1 1/2 c. half-and-half
- 3 c. sugar
- 3 TBSP. light corn syrup
- 2 tsp. vanilla extract
- 1 1/2 c. roughly chopped pecans

Direction

- Line an 8-inch square baking pan with parchment paper that extends over the sides. Coat the paper with 1 TBSP. of the butter; set aside.
- In a 3-quart heavy-bottomed saucepan over low heat, cook the maple syrup, half-and-half, sugar, corn syrup, and salt until the sugar is dissolved (about 5 minutes), stirring constantly with a long-handled wooden spoon.
- Bring the mixture to a boil over medium heat, then brush down the sides of the pan with a pastry brush dipped in warm water to prevent the sugar from crystallizing. Place candy thermometer in the pan and cook the mixture without stirring until it registers 238 degrees F on the thermometer (about 15 minutes).
- Remove the pan from the heat, remove the thermometer from the pan, and place the thermometer in warm water to cool. Sprinkle a large baking sheet with high sides with cold water and immediately pour the mixture onto the baking sheet. Do not scrape the bottom of the pan.
- Dot the surface of the mixture with the remaining 3 TBSP. butter. Let the mixture cool on the baking sheet until it registers 110 degrees F on the thermometer, about 15 - 20 minutes.
- Transfer the mixture to the bowl of a stand mixer, add the vanilla, and with the paddle attachment, beat the mixture until it thickens and loses its shine (5 to 10 minutes).
- Add the pecans and mix until they are blended in, about 30 seconds.
- Turn the fudge into the prepared pan. Use your fingertips to even the top and to press the fudge into the corners of the pan. Place the pan of fudge on a cooling rack and let it set completely at room temperature, 1 to 2 hours.
- Remove the fudge from the pan by lifting out the parchment paper. Invert the fudge onto a cutting board, peel the paper off the back of the fudge, and reinvert the fudge. With a large chef's knife, cut the fudge evenly into 1-inch squares.
- To store, layer fudge between waxed paper in an airtight container for up to 10 days at room temperature or 1 month in the refrigerator. The fudge is best served at room temperature.

104. Marilyns Rocky Road Heaven Recipe

Serving: 12 | Prep: | Cook: 2mins | Ready in:

Ingredients

- 1 cup dark chocolate Candy Coating Disks
- 1 cup Mini-Colored fruit Flavored marshmallows
- 1/4 cup Chopped pecans
- 1/4 cup semi-sweet chocolate chips

Direction

- Line a cookie sheet with waxed paper.
- Put chocolate coating disks into micro-wave safe bowl or pot. Melt on HIGH for 30 seconds. Stir. Repeat till the chocolate is melted.
- While chocolate is melting, put rest of ingredients in lrg. bowl and when chocolate coating is ready, pour it over and mix, making sure everything is well coated, but not overly.
- Drop by teaspoonfuls onto waxed paper. Refrigerate for 15 mins. or until set and shiny. (To make these fancier, instead of dropping onto waxed paper, drop into candy cups placed onto cookie sheet with sides and then refrigerate as above.)
- These are addictive!!! Hubby & I are really enjoying them & I hope you will enjoy too!

105. Marshmallow Nut Truffles Recipe

Serving: 40 | Prep: | Cook: 5mins | Ready in:

Ingredients

- 1 7-ounce jar marshmallow creme
- 1/3 cup butter, softened
- 1/4 teaspoon almond extract or vanilla*
- 1/4 teaspoon salt
- 3 cups powdered sugar
- toasted whole almonds, toasted pecan halves, toasted macadamia nuts, toasted hazelnuts (filberts), quartered pitted dates, and/or dried cherries
- powdered sugar
- 8 ounces semisweet chocolate squares, chopped**
- 1 tablespoon shortening
- Finely chopped toasted nuts, toasted coconut, or candy sprinkles
- White baking chocolate, melted

Direction

- 1. Line a large baking sheet with waxed paper; butter the paper. Set aside. In a large bowl, combine marshmallow crème, butter, almond extract, and salt. Beat with an electric mixer until smooth. Gradually add the 3 cups powdered sugar, beating until well mixed. Cover and chill about 1 hour or until mixture is easy to handle.
- 2. Lightly dust your hands with additional powdered sugar; shape marshmallow mixture into 1-inch balls, forming the mixture around a whole almond, pecan half, macadamia nut, hazelnut (filbert), date piece, or dried cherry (you may need more marshmallow mixture to completely cover the pecan halves and almonds). Place balls on prepared baking sheet. Cover lightly; freeze for 20 minutes.
- 3. Meanwhile, in a small saucepan, combine semisweet chocolate and shortening. Heat and stir over low heat until melted and smooth. Remove from heat.
- 4. Line another large baking sheet with waxed paper; set aside. Remove balls, a few at a time, from the freezer; dip balls in chocolate and use a fork to lift balls out of chocolate, drawing the fork across the rim of the saucepan to remove excess chocolate. Place balls on waxed-paper-lined baking sheet. Immediately sprinkle tops with finely chopped nuts, toasted coconut, or candy sprinkles. Let stand at room temperature about 15 minutes or until completely set. If desired, drizzle truffles with melted white chocolate.
- Makes about 40 truffles.
- Test Kitchen Tip
- If you prefer, omit the almond extract or vanilla and add 1 tablespoon desired flavored liqueur (such as raspberry or orange) to the marshmallow mixture; increase the 3 cups powdered sugar to 3-1/4 cups.
- Test Kitchen Tip
- You may use 8 ounces vanilla-flavor candy coating instead of (or in addition to) the semisweet chocolate. If using both, in separate small saucepans, combine the candy coating or semisweet chocolate with the shortening; melt, dip, and decorate truffles as directed. (You

will have leftover melted candy coating and chocolate, but use 8 ounces of each so you get enough depth to dip truffles.) If desired, drizzle white-coated truffles with melted semisweet chocolate.
- TO STORE
- Layer truffles between pieces of waxed paper in an airtight container; cover. Store in the refrigerator for up to 1 week or freeze for up to 3 months.

106. Martha Washington Balls Recipe

Serving: 20 | Prep: | Cook: 5mins | Ready in:

Ingredients

- 2 cups coconut
- 2 cups chopped pecans
- 1 can condensed milk
- 2 1/2 cups powdered sugar
- 1 teaspoon vanilla
- 1 6oz package chocolate chips
- 1/2 bar parafin

Direction

- Mix all ingredients together. Let chill for about an hour.
- Then roll mixture into balls about the size of between nickels and quarters, not to small but not too big. Rechill.
- Dipping sauce:
- Melt chocolate chips and paraffin in double boiler.
- Dip each round ball into chocolate and set on wax paper to harden.
- Take a toothpick and stick in balls to dip. This makes it easier.

107. Mexican Orange Candy Recipe

Serving: 12 | Prep: | Cook: 30mins | Ready in:

Ingredients

- 3 cups granulated sugar
- 1-1/2 cups scalded milk
- 1 cup pecans
- Granted rind of 2 oranges
- 1/2 cup unsalted butter

Direction

- Melt 1 cup sugar in large pan over medium heat while milk is scalding in another saucepan.
- When sugar is melted and a golden brown color add hot milk all at once stirring constantly.
- Add remaining sugar and keep stirring until dissolved.
- Cook until it forms a hard ball in water or use a candy thermometer.
- Just before it is done add grated orange rind, butter and nuts.
- Remove from heat and beat until creamy.
- Pour into a buttered 9" square pan to cool.
- Cut into squares when cooled.

108. Mexican Pralines Recipe

Serving: 24 | Prep: | Cook: 20mins | Ready in:

Ingredients

- 2 1/2 cups sugar
- 1 can (5.33) evaporated milk
- 2 tablespoons white Karo syrup
- 2 tablespoons butter
- 2 cups pecans, chopped

Direction

- Mix first 4 ingredients in a saucepan and bring to a boil.
- Add pecans and cook to soft ball candy stage (238 degrees)
- Remove from heat.
- Beat until creamy.
- Drop by teaspoons on waxed paper.

109. Microwave Fudge Recipe

Serving: 8 | Prep: | Cook: 10mins | Ready in:

Ingredients

- 3-2/3 cups confectioners' sugar
- 1/2 cup cocoa
- 1/4 cup milk
- 1/2 cup butter
- 1 tablespoon vanilla
- 1/2 cup chopped pecans, optional

Direction

- Combine and cook sugar, cocoa, milk and butter on high power until butter is melted.
- Stir until smooth.
- Blend in vanilla and pecans.
- Spread into a buttered 8-inch square pan.
- Chill then cut in squares.

110. Microwave Praline Recipe

Serving: 812 | Prep: | Cook: 25mins | Ready in:

Ingredients

- 1-1/2 cups sugar
- 1 can condensed milk
- 1 stick of butter softened
- 1 Tsp vanilla extract
- 1-1/2 cup pecans chopped

Direction

- Line counter top with waxed paper (about 2-1/2 feet)
- Place first three ingredients in a 3-quart-microwave safe glass bowl.
- Microwave on high for 2-minute intervals x 4 (8 min total). Each time take out and stir.
- Then stir in pecans and vanilla and place back in microwave for 3 minutes. Candy should be the consistency and color of peanut butter.
- Stir, place back in microwave for 2 minutes.
- Drop candy by tablespoons onto waxed paper. Allow to cool and harden. ENJOY!

111. Microwave Pralines 1 Recipe

Serving: 10 | Prep: | Cook: 12mins | Ready in:

Ingredients

- 1 1/2 cups firmly packed light brown sugar
- 2/3 cup evaporated milk
- 1/8 tsp. salt
- 2 Tbsp. butter or margarine
- 1 1/2 cup pecan halves
- 1/2 tsp. vanilla extract

Direction

- Combine sugar, milk and salt in a 3 quart casserole bowl; mix well.
- Add butter and microwave on high for 10 to 12 minutes. Check to make sure mixture has reached the soft ball stage. Add pecans and vanilla.
- Cool slightly. Drop by tablespoons onto wax paper to set up.

112. Microwave Sugar Spiced Pecans Recipe

Serving: 8 | Prep: | Cook: 67mins | Ready in:

Ingredients

- 1 cup sugar
- 1/3 cup evaporated milk
- 1/2 teaspoon cinnamon
- 1 1/2 tablespoons butter
- 1 1/2 cups pecan halves
- 1/2 teaspoon vanilla extract

Direction

- Mix all but pecans and vanilla extract in a LARGE microwave safe bowl. (I use an 8-qt. measuring cup) The mixture really boils up high once it's hot.
- Microwave on high for 6 or 7 minutes, stirring every 2 or 3 minutes. You can usually tell it's getting close to the soft ball stage when it tends to stop bubbling and rising as it was earlier.
- Remove from microwave, stir in nuts and vanilla extract. It usually hardens up really quick for me, but if you feel it's too runny of a mixture you can beat it with a spoon for a few seconds.
- Drop quickly onto wax paper, separating the halves as much as possible.
- Allow to cool completely and store in air tight containers or jars.

113. Microwave Toffee Recipe

Serving: 4 | Prep: | Cook: 8mins | Ready in:

Ingredients

- 1 cup chopped pecans or toasted almonds
- 1 cup sugar
- 1/4 cup water
- 1 stick of regular salted butter
- 1/2 cup semi-sweet chocolate morsels

Direction

- Sprinkle your chopped nuts over either a silicone pad or a 12 inch piece of Release aluminum foil. (This foil is great to use!)
- Sprinkle the nuts in a circle about 10 inches length, keeping the nut pieces close together. You can also use a 9 inch pan, well-buttered!
- In a microwave-proof glass bowl, add the water, butter and sugar.
- Cook on high for seven minutes.
- Do not stop and stir your mixture. Just let it cook!
- If the mixture in the bowl is not a caramel-ish, lightly brown color, cook for one minute more.
- Remove bowl from microwave and pour the sugar mixture directly over the nuts.
- Using a rubber spatula, push the nuts on the sides into the edges of the mixture before it cools so that you don't waste nuts that are not attached to the candy.
- Quickly sprinkle your chocolate chips over the top of the candy and let it melt there for about 2 minutes.
- Spread the melting chips over the top of your toffee.
- I like to sprinkle this with extra nuts.
- Let the toffee cool completely.
- Break into pieces and serve!

114. Millionaires Recipe

Serving: 48 | Prep: | Cook: 30mins | Ready in:

Ingredients

- 14oz. pk. caramels, unwrapped
- 2tbs. milk
- 2c. chopped pecans
- 10oz. pk. milk chocolate mini kisses

Direction

- Combine caramels and milk in a heavy saucepan; cook mixture over low heat, stirring constantly, until smooth.
- Stir in pecans, and drop by teaspoonfuls onto buttered baking sheets. Let stand until firm.
- Microwave milk chocolates in a 1 quart microwave-safe bowl at High 1 minute or until melted, stirring once.
- Dip caramel candies into melted chocolate, allowing excess to drip; place on buttered baking sheets. Let candy stand until firm.

115. Missouri Colonels Recipe

Serving: 8 | Prep: | Cook: | Ready in:

Ingredients

- 4 cups sifted confectioners' sugar, divided
- 1 cup finely chopped pecans
- 1/2 cup butter, softened
- 1/4 cup green creme de menthe
- 1 (6 ounce) package semisweet chocolate pieces (1 cup)
- 1 teaspoon shortening

Direction

- In large mixing bowl, beat together 2 cups of the confectioners' sugar, the pecans, butter and crème de menthe. Beat or stir in remaining confectioners' sugar. Cover and chill mixture for 1 hour or until firm.
- Shape into 1-inch balls. Place balls on a foil- or wax paper-lined baking sheet. Chill for 15 minutes.
- In a small, heavy saucepan, heat chocolate pieces and shortening over very low heat, stirring constantly, until chocolate melts. Dip one side of each of the chilled balls into melted chocolate. Return to baking sheet. Chill until set.
- Makes about 60 candies.
- NOTE: For a non-alcoholic candy, use 1/4 cup corn syrup, 1/4 teaspoon peppermint extract and a few drops green food coloring for crème de menthe.
- Make-Ahead Tip: Prepare candies as above. Cover and store in refrigerator for up to 1 week. Or freeze candies in a freezer container for up to 3 months.

116. Moms Secret Fudge Recipe Recipe

Serving: 15 | Prep: | Cook: 20mins | Ready in:

Ingredients

- 1 king size Hershey chocolate Bar.... (7 - 8 oz.)
- 12 oz. bag of Nestle's chocolate Dots --- mini semi sweet chocolate chips
- 1 1/2 cups walnuts -chopped
- 1/2 cup pecans - chopped
- 1/4 cup almonds - chopped
- 1 jar (7-8 oz.) Marshmellow Fluff
- ....
- 1/3 cup butter
- 1 cup evaporated milk
- 4 1/2 cups superfine sugar
- extra butter

Direction

- In a large heavy bowl that can stand heat.
- Break up Hershey Bar into pieces.
- Add chocolate dots on top.
- Then add the nuts.
- And top with marshmallow fluff.
- Put in a warm spot so the chocolate starts to soften.
- ....
- In a heavy pan, butter the sides and bottom of the pan heavily.
- Put in 1/3 cup of butter and the evaporated milk.
- Heat until warm.
- Slowly add the sugar. Stir after each addition.

- Make sure the dry sugar does not touch the sides of the pan.
- Don't stir too hard, you don't want the sugar mixture all over the sides of the pan.
- Heat slowly until the sugar is dissolved keep stirring.
- DON'T scrap the sides of the pan.
- The turn the heat up to medium.
- Using a candy thermometer bring temperature to 225-228' F.
- Stir mixture to keep from burning.
- Pour hot sugar mixture over chocolate mixture in the bowl.
- DO NOT scrape the pot out.
- Use a new spoon and blend the together as quickly as possible.
- DON"T over mix. There will be some streaks of the fluff that's ok.
- Spread mixture on a well-buttered jelly roll pan. (Large spatula works).
- Work quickly. This fudge sets up very fast.
- Cover tightly with plastic wrap and then foil.
- Put in a cold spot for 4 hours. Cut into pieces.
- ....
- Keep wrapped tightly. This fudge dries out very fast.

117. My Favorite Fudge Recipe

Serving: 12 | Prep: | Cook: 20mins | Ready in:

Ingredients

- 2 Cups Granulated sugar
- 1/4 Cup of Hershey's Coca
- Small Pinch of salt
- 1 Cup of Half and Half
- 1 Tbsp. white Karo syrup
- 2 Tbsp. butter
- 1 Tsp. vanilla
- 1/4 Cup Chopped Chopped pecans
- 1/4 Cup Chopped Red candied cherries

Direction

- Combine All Ingredients In A 2 Qt. Heavy Metal Saucepan. Stir Until All Lumps Are Dissolved. Cook and stir on Medium High until All Sugar is dissolved and Mixture Feels Smooth.
- When Candy Begins to Boil, Reduce Heat to Low and Stop Stirring.
- Continue Cooking to the Soft Ball Stage, Remove from heat and add Butter. When Fudge Is Cool to the Touch, Add Vanilla and Beat Until It Begins to Solidify.
- Quickly Add Chopped Pecans and Cherries and Transfer to An 8 x 8 Buttered Dish.
- Let Set for 25 Minutes and Then Cut Into Squares, Cover and Store in a Cool Place.

118. My Favorite Fudge Recipe

Serving: 50 | Prep: | Cook: 4mins | Ready in:

Ingredients

- 6 cps sugar
- 3 sticks butter (do not use margarine)
- 1 1/2 cp half and half
- 3 8 oz bags dove dark chocolate promises
- 1 large jar marshmallow cream
- 1 1/2 cp chopped pecans
- 1 tbs vanilla
- 1/4 tsp salt

Direction

- Prepare 9x13 pan by lining with aluminum foil, bringing it up the sides of the pan.
- Unwrap dove pieces.
- Place sugar, butter, half and half and salt in large heavy pan.
- On medium heat gently bring to a hard boil stirring all the time.
- Boil for 4 minutes stirring all the time to prevent scorching.

- Turn off heat and add chocolate and marshmallow cream.
- Let stand five minutes to melt the chocolate.
- Add vanilla and stir till completely blended.
- Add pecans and stir in.
- Pour into prepared pan.
- Cool completely.
- Remove from pan and cut into one inch squares.
- Makes about 5 lbs. fudge.
- I wrap mine individually in waxed paper and store in a jar with a lid. Keeps for a long time if someone doesn't eat them all.
- Enjoy and everyone have a Merry Christmas or whatever you celebrate.

119. My First Chocolate Fudge Recipe

Serving: 24 | Prep: | Cook: 20mins | Ready in:

Ingredients

- 4-1/2. cups granulate sugar
- 12 oz. can evaporated milk
- 1/4 lb. butter
- 1 jar marshmallow creme
- 12 oz. semi-sweet chocolate chips
- 12 oz. milk chocolate bar
- 2 cups Chopped pecans or walnuts
- Note: I have added 1 cup miniature marshmallows and 1/2 cup pecans/walnuts to this recipe and it's great!
- 2 tsp. vanilla

Direction

- Cook sugar, milk, and butter to soft ball stage - 234 degrees on candy thermometer, stirring constantly.
- Remove from heat and add the remaining ingredients.
- Stir quickly and thoroughly to blend.
- Pour into a large lightly buttered baking pan or dish

- Cool then cut into squares and store in the refrigerator.

120. My Homemade Toffee Recipe

Serving: 10 | Prep: | Cook: 15mins | Ready in:

Ingredients

- 1 Cup Granulated sugar
- 1 Cup butter (2 Sticks)
- 1/4 Cup water
- 4 Hershey Bars
- 1/2 Cup Finely Chopped pecans (I Put Mine In A Ziplock and Beat Them Up with the Bottom of A Heavy Glass or A Mallet)

Direction

- Combine First Three (3) Ingredients in A Heavy Skillet. Stirring Constantly, Cook Over High Heat Until Mixture Turns to A Tan Color and Begins to Smoke.
- Quickly Pour Onto A Cookie Sheet and Cool Slightly. Break Chocolate Into Squares and Scatter Over Hot Toffee, Spreading Smoothly with A Knife While It Melts. Top with the Finely Chopped Pecans. Let Cool Completely, Break Into Chunks and Store in An Air Tight Container.

121. My Tutti Frutti Fudge Recipe

Serving: 24 | Prep: | Cook: 10mins | Ready in:

Ingredients

- 18 oz. good quality semi-sweet chocolate chips
- 8 oz. whole marshmallows, cut up in bite size pieces

- 2 cups coarse chopped nuts (walnuts, pecans, macadamias etc.)
- 1 8 oz. jar marachino cherries chopped and drained well
- 1 tsp. pure vanilla extract
- 1/2 cup flaked coconut (optional)
- 1 can evaporated (not condensed) milk
- 2 sticks butter or margarine
- 4 1/2 cups white granulated sugar

Direction

- Prepare on a dry day: (It sets up better)
- Butter the bottom of a 9 x 13 inch oblong pan.
- In a large bowl combine the chocolate chips, cherries, nuts and cut up marshmallows and set aside.
- In a large heavy (good quality) saucepan melt butter over low heat.
- Add and stir in sugar and milk.
- Increase heat to medium and stir constantly until mixture comes to a boil.
- Once a rolling boil, boil 10 minutes only stirring now and then.
- After the 10 minutes pour the mixture over the reserved chocolate, nuts, cherries and marshmallows stirring to melt chocolate but leave marshmallows partially unmelted.
- Stir in vanilla.
- Pour mixture into the buttered pan.
- Sprinkle the coconut on top.
- Cool completely at room temperature.
- Chill and cut.
- Note: this fudge recipe is very versatile.
- You may stir coconut into mixture if desired or even omit it.
- You may use raisins instead of nuts or substitute candied pineapple for the cherries etc.

122. NUTTY SWEET CARAMELS Recipe

Serving: 60 | Prep: | Cook: 30mins | Ready in:

Ingredients

- 2/3 cup pecans
- 2 cups granulated sugar
- 1 stick (1/2 cup) butter
- 2 cups whipping cream
- 3/4 cup light corn syrup

Direction

- Toast pecans on cookie sheet in 350°F oven for about 8 minutes or until you can smell them.
- Cool; chop fine with sharp knife. You can put in a zip lock bag, cover with a towel and let kids hit them.
- Butter the inside of an 8-inch square glass baking dish.
- Sprinkle pecans evenly over bottom of dish; set aside.
- In a heavy 3-quart saucepan, combine sugar, butter, whipping cream and syrup.
- Bring to a boil over medium heat, stirring constantly.
- Place candy thermometer in pan.
- Cook, stirring frequently, until temperature reaches 245°F or a tablespoon of mixture dropped into very cold water forms a firm ball when handled. (It is important to stir mixture to prevent sticking.)
- DO NOT LET KIDS HANDLE HOT PAN WITH CANDY.
- I never time it, I go by the thermometer, times above are a guess.
- Pour caramel over pecans.
- Cool at room temperature for about 1 hour.
- Run knife around dish edges; invert over cutting surface using edge of knife to help release caramel.
- Cut into small squares with a WET, sharp knife using a sawing motion. You might have to rewet knife more than once.
- Wrap individually in plastic wrap or wax paper when cooled completely.

123. New Orleans Pralines Recipe

Serving: 8 | Prep: | Cook: 20mins | Ready in:

Ingredients

- 1 cup sugar
- 1 cup brown sugar
- 3 Tablespoons butter
- 2/3 cup sweetened condensed milk
- 1 1/2 Tablespoons vanilla
- 1- 1 1/2 cup pecan pieces

Direction

- Mix first 4 ingredients together. Cook and stir for 20 minutes on med high. Add vanilla and pecans. Drop by spoonful on wax paper.

124. No Bake Cocoa Bourbon Balls Recipe

Serving: 12 | Prep: | Cook: | Ready in:

Ingredients

- 1 cup vanilla wafers crushed fine
- 1 cup powdered sugar
- 1 cup chopped pecans
- 2 tablespoons cocoa
- 2 tablespoons light corn syrup
- 1/4 cup bourbon
- Granulated sugar

Direction

- Stir together crumbs, confectioners' sugar, pecans and cocoa then add corn syrup and bourbon.
- Mix well and with wet hands shape into 1" balls then roll in granulated sugar.

125. Nutty Caramels Recipe

Serving: 24 | Prep: | Cook: 30mins | Ready in:

Ingredients

- 3/4 cup pecans, chopped
- 2 cups heavy cream
- 1 cup brown sugar
- 1 cup granulated sugar
- 1 cup light corn syrup
- 1/4 cup butter
- 1/4 tsp salt
- 1 tsp vanilla

Direction

- Prepare an 8-inch square baking pan by lining it with aluminum foil.
- 2. Lightly heat the heavy cream until warm. You can place it in the microwave for 20-30 seconds, or put it on the stove in a small saucepan.
- 3. Mix together 1 cup of warm cream, the sugar, and the corn syrup in a large saucepan over medium heat. Bring to a boil and slowly pour in the remaining cream.
- 4. Continue heating the mixture until it comes to 230 degrees.
- 5. Add the butter in small chunks, stirring to encourage melting. Allow the mixture to reach 245 degrees (firm ball stage).
- 6. Remove from heat and stir in pecans, vanilla and salt.
- 7. Pour into the prepared pan, and allow to fully set at room temperature.

126. Nutty Heavenly Hash Recipe

Serving: 12 | Prep: | Cook: 20mins | Ready in:

Ingredients

- 2 cups sugar

- 1 tablespoon butter
- 1/2 cup blanched and roasted almonds
- 2 tablespoons marshmallow cream
- 1 teaspoon vanilla
- 1/2 cup chopped pecans
- 4 tablespoons grated unsweetened chocolate
- 24 marshmallows
- 1 cup cream

Direction

- Combine chocolate and sugar then add cream and butter.
- Boil to soft ball stage then remove from fire.
- Add marshmallow cream, nuts and flavoring.
- Beat until mixture begins to thicken.
- Place marshmallows on well-buttered dish evenly.
- Pour mixture over marshmallows then allow to cool and cut in squares.

127. Old Fashion Brown Sugar Fudge Recipe

Serving: 24 | Prep: | Cook: | Ready in:

Ingredients

- 2 cups brown sugar
- 1 cup granulated sugar
- 1 cup evaporated milk
- 1/2 cup butter
- 1 teaspoon vanilla
- 1 cup chopped pecans or walnuts

Direction

- Combine sugars, milk, and butter. Cook, stirring occasionally, to soft-ball stage, or 238° on a candy thermometer. Add vanilla and let cool to lukewarm. Beat with wooden spoon until mixture loses its gloss; stir in nuts. Pour into a buttered 8-inch pan or pie plate.
- Cool brown sugar fudge until firm and cut into squares.

128. Old Fashioned Date Confection Recipe

Serving: 12 | Prep: | Cook: 20mins | Ready in:

Ingredients

- 2 cups sugar
- 1 cup whole milk
- 2 tablespoons butter
- 1-1/2 cups chopped dates
- 1 cup chopped pecans

Direction

- Combine the sugar, milk and butter in a heavy saucepan.
- Stirring occasionally, cook over medium heat to soft ball stage (238°F on candy thermometer).
- Stir the dates and pecans into the syrup and continue cooking until dates are dissolved and mixture reaches firm ball stage (248°F on candy thermometer).
- Remove from heat and allow to cool.
- Pour mixture out onto clean, damp dishtowels or tea towels and shape into 2-inch diameter rolls.
- Chill until firm.
- Slice in half-inch slices.

129. Orange Chocolate Meltaways Recipe

Serving: 0 | Prep: | Cook: 40mins | Ready in:

Ingredients

- 1 package (11 ounces) chocolate chips
- 1 cup (6 ounces) milk chocolate chips
- 3/4 cup heavy whipping cream

- 1 teaspoon grated orange peel
- 2 1/2 teaspoons orange extract
- 1 1/2 cups finely chopped toasted pecans
- chocolate for coating

Direction

1. Put the chocolate chips in a bowl and set aside, in a pan bring the cream and orange peel to a gentle boil and pour over chips let stand for one minute and then whisk until smooth cover and chill for 35 minutes or until mixture begins to thicken.
2. Beat the mixture for 10-15 seconds or just until it lightens in color (but do not overbeat) place rounded teaspoons of mixture on wax paper lined baking sheet.
3. Gentle shape into balls and roll some in nuts and then melt some chocolate and dip the rest and store them in an airtight container in the fridge.

130. Orange Juice Balls Recipe

Serving: 24 | Prep: | Cook: 10mins | Ready in:

Ingredients

- 1 12 oz. box vanilla wafers crushed
- 1 cups confectioners sugar
- 1/4 cup melted butter or margarine
- 1 6 oz. can frozen orange juice
- 3/4 cups chopped nuts (I use pecans)
- Extra confectioner's sugar

Direction

- Blend first 5 ingredients well.
- Make into walnut size balls
- Roll in the confectioner's sugar
- Refrigerate well (about 2-4 hours)
- Makes 4 dozen balls.
- Enjoy.

131. Orange Pecans Recipe

Serving: 8 | Prep: | Cook: 25mins | Ready in:

Ingredients

- 1 cup of sugar
- juice of two oranges
- grated rind of one orange
- 1 teaspoon of cayenne pepper (more if you dare)
- or substitute a chipotle powder for a smokier kick
- generous pinch of salt
- 1 lb. of shelled pecan halves

Direction

- Mix sugar, juice and rind in a saucepan.
- Bring to a boil.
- Reduce heat.
- Cook slowly 15 minutes.
- Remove from heat, stir in pepper, salt and pecans.
- Stir.
- When well coated, drop from tip of spoon onto greased cookie sheet or wax paper.
- Cool.
- Store in airtight container.

132. PECAN CLUSTERS Recipe

Serving: 0 | Prep: | Cook: | Ready in:

Ingredients

- 3 pounds pecans
- 1-2 tablespoons real butter
- 2 12 ounce packages chocolate chips
- 1 package, plus 4 from another package almond bark

Direction

- In a heavy skillet, melt butter.
- Add pecans
- Stir until pecans get toasty; do not burn
- Drain on paper towel until cool.
- Melt chips and almond bark in a double pan over hot water.
- When melted add pecans, stir to mix.
- Let set for about 10 minutes.
- Drop by tablespoons on waxed paper
- Let set, store in a very cool place.
- Yummmmy!

133. PECAN DELIGHTS Recipe

Serving: 36 | Prep: | Cook: 15mins | Ready in:

Ingredients

- Ingredients:
- 2 ¼ cups packed brown sugar
- 1 cup butter or margarine
- 1 cup light corn syrup
- 1/8 tsp. salt
- 1 can (14-oz) sweetened condensed milk
- 1 tsp. vanilla extract
- 1 ½ pounds whole pecans
- 1 cup (6-oz) semisweet chocolate chips
- 1 cup (6-oz) milk chocolate chips
- 2 Tbs. shortening

Direction

- In a large saucepan, combine the first four ingredients. Cook over medium heat until al sugar is dissolved. Gradually add candy thermometer reads 248 (firm-ball stage). Remove from the heat; stir in vanilla until blended. Fold in the pecans. Drop by tablespoonful onto a waxed paper-lined cookie sheet. Chill until firm. Melt chocolate chips and shortening in a microwave-safe bowl or double boiler. Drizzle over each cluster. Cool.

134. POOR MAN TURTLES Recipe

Serving: 15 | Prep: | Cook: 5mins | Ready in:

Ingredients

- Minature pretzels
- Rolo Candy
- pecan halves

Direction

- Preheat oven to 250°
- Line a cookie sheet with foil.
- Put pretzels on foil.
- Put 1 Rolo candy on top of each pretzel.
- Put in a preheated oven for 5 minutes.
- Remove from oven and immediately put one pecan half on top of Rolo candy mashing it down to fill the pretzel.
- Refrigerate until set. Store in a tight sealing dish.

135. PRETZEL BITES Recipe

Serving: 30 | Prep: | Cook: 7mins | Ready in:

Ingredients

- 1 BAG pretzel TWISTS
- 1 BAG ROLO candies
- 1 BAG pecan halves

Direction

- Place the pretzel twist on a cookie sheet
- Top with a roll candy
- Place in a 350° oven until soft
- Remove from the oven and place a pecan halve on each top while still hot

- Let cool and serve

136. Pa & Ma's Wonderful Holiday Fudge Recipe

Serving: 30 | Prep: | Cook: 1hours | Ready in:

Ingredients

- 1 stick butter.
- 4-1/2 cups sugar.
- 1 12 oz. can evaporated milk.
- 1 12 oz. package milk chocolate.
- 1 12 oz. package chocolate chips.
- 2 oz. unsweetened chocolate squares, broken apart.
- 1 tablespoon vanilla.
- 1/2 pound Kraft miniature marshmallows.
- 2 cups broken walnuts, or pecans.

Direction

- 1. Prepare the Kraft marshmallows, nuts of choice, vanilla, and chocolates, set aside.
- 2. Set a good digital timer to 6-1/2 minutes, set aside.
- 3. Butter a 10 X 15 inch jelly roll pan, set aside.
- 4. In a 10 inch Dutch oven, over medium heat, cook the first three ingredients, stirring well.
- 5. When the mixture begins to boil, start the timer and cook 6-1/2 minutes.
- 6. Do not remove cover until cooking time is over. Immediately remove from heat.
- 7. Add Kraft marshmallows, and stir well. Add chocolates, 1 at a time stirring well.
- 8. Add vanilla, stirring well, then add nuts, and mix until well blended.
- 9. Pour into buttered jelly roll pan and spread out evenly. Cover, cool, cut, and enjoy.

137. Peanut Brittle Wanda Recipe

Serving: 15 | Prep: | Cook: 15mins | Ready in:

Ingredients

- 1/2 cup water
- 2 cups sugar
- 1 cup white Karo syrup
- 2 cups raw peanuts or pecans
- 2 tsp baking soda
- 2 Tbls butter
- 1 tsp vanilla

Direction

- Bring water to boil. Add sugar & karo stirring until dissolved.
- Boil without stirring for 15 minutes or until temperature reaches 230 degrees.
- Add nuts and cook over low heat until Karo turns a golden brown.
- Take from fire. Add butter, soda and vanilla stirring just enough to mix.
- Spread on large cookie sheet that has been well buttered.
- Cool. Break into pieces.

138. Peanut Brittle Ice Cream Pie With Chocolate Sauce Recipe

Serving: 1 | Prep: | Cook: 15mins | Ready in:

Ingredients

- See Directions.

Direction

- Crust
- 7 oz (1 pkg) coconut
- 1/2 cup pecans, chopped
- 2 tablespoons all purpose flour

- 1/2 stick margarine, melted
- Mix flour with coconut and pecans; add melted margarine and stir. Pat into 10-inch pie plate. Bake for 10-20 minutes, or until lightly browned at 350 degrees.
- Filling
- 1/2 gallon vanilla ice cream
- 1/2-3/4 cup crushed peanut brittle
- Mix softened ice cream and peanut brittle. Place into cooled pie shell for at least 6 hours.
- Fudge sauce
- 1/2 cup cocoa
- 1 cup granulated sugar
- 1 cup light corn syrup
- 4 tablespoons butter or margarine
- 4 tablespoons light cream
- 1/4 tsp salt
- 1 tsp vanilla
- Mix first five ingredients in sauce pan. Bring to boil, boiling for three minutes, stirring constantly. Remove from heat, add salt and vanilla. Cool and drizzle over whipped cream, atop pie. All steps may be done before presentation.

139. Peanut Buttery Chocolate Balls Recipe

Serving: 70 | Prep: | Cook: 60mins | Ready in:

Ingredients

- 2 sticks of margarine
- 1 box powdered sugar
- 1/2 qt. crunchy peanut butter
- 1/2 cup ground pecans
- 8 oz. chocolate chips
- 1/2 block of parafin wax

Direction

- Mix softened margarine, powdered sugar, peanut butter, and pecans in a large mixing bowl with a spoon (or hands).
- Melt chocolate and paraffin wax in a double broiler until smooth.
- Mold peanut butter mixture into one inch balls, dip into chocolate and wax mixture, being sure to cover all surface.
- Place on wax-covered cookie sheet, and chill in the fridge for at least 1 hour.
- ENJOY!

140. Pecan Caramel Spiders Recipe

Serving: 30 | Prep: | Cook: 30mins | Ready in:

Ingredients

- 1 1/2 cups toasted pecans
- 1 cup heavy cream
- 1 cup granulated sugar
- 1/2 cup light corn syrup
- 1 teaspoon vanilla extract
- 2 tablespoons unsalted butter, in pieces
- 1/4 teaspoon salt
- 5 ounces thin black licorice strands, cut into 2-inch pieces
- 6 ounces semisweet chocolate, chopped
- 4 ounces milk chocolate, chopped
- chocolate curls or jimmies, optional

Direction

- Line 2 baking sheets with waxed paper and lightly spray with non-stick spray.
- Mound 30 small clusters of pecans, about 3 or 4 pecans each, spaced a couple inches apart on the pan.
- Make caramel: Warm the cream over low heat and keep warm while you cook the sugar.
- Put the sugar and corn syrup and in a deep, heavy-bottomed large saucepan.
- Cook over medium heat, stirring occasionally until the sugar dissolves.
- Stop stirring, raise heat to medium-high, and simmer until the sugar reaches the hard crack

stage, or 305 degrees F on a candy thermometer, about 7 minutes.
- Whisk the butter and salt into the sugar mixture.
- Gradually pour in the cream and vanilla taking care since the mixture will bubble up.
- Reduce the heat to medium and continue to cook, stirring occasionally, until the sugar reaches soft ball stage, 240 degrees F on the thermometer, about 5 minutes more.
- Immediately remove from the heat and cool for a minute.
- Ladle a couple tablespoons of warm caramel over some of the nut clusters, to make the spider bodies.
- Then press 6 pieces of licorice into the warm caramel to make the legs.
- Repeat with the remaining caramel and licorice.
- (It's helpful to have an extra hand here, since the caramel can set quickly.
- If caramel hardens, warm over very low heat.)
- Let spiders cool 15 minutes.
- ~
- Meanwhile, put the chocolates in a medium heatproof bowl.
- Bring a saucepan filled with 1-inch or so of water to a very slow simmer; set the bowl over, but not touching, the water.
- Stir the chocolate occasionally until melted and smooth.
- (Alternatively, put the chocolate in a medium microwave-safe bowl. Melt at 50 percent power in the microwave until soft, about 1 minute. Stir, and continue heat until completely melted, 2 to 3 minutes more.)
- ~
- Spoon about 1 tablespoon of melted chocolate on top of each spider.
- Sprinkle with jimmies or chocolate curls, if desired.
- Let cool until firm.
- ~
- Copyright 2007 Television Food Network, G.P. All rights reserved

141. Pecan Caramel Spiders Recipe

Serving: 30 | Prep: | Cook: 30mins | Ready in:

Ingredients

- 1 1/2 cups toasted pecans
- 1 cup heavy cream
- 1 cup granulated sugar
- 1/2 cup light corn syrup
- 1 teaspoon vanilla extract
- 2 tablespoons unsalted butter, in pieces
- 1/4 teaspoon salt
- 5 ounces thin black licorice strands, cut into 2-inch pieces
- 6 ounces semisweet chocolate, chopped
- 4 ounces milk chocolate, chopped
- chocolate curls or jimmies, optional
- Directions:
- Line 2 baking sheets with waxed paper and lightly spray with
- nonstick spray.
- Mound 30 small clusters of pecans, about 3 or 4 pecans each, spaced a
- couple inches apart on the pan.
- Make caramel: Warm the cream over low heat and keep warm while you
- cook the sugar.
- Put the sugar and corn syrup and in a deep, heavy-bottomed large
- saucepan.
- Cook over medium heat, stirring occasionally until the sugar
- dissolves.
- Stop stirring, raise heat to medium-high, and simmer until the sugar
- reaches the hard crack stage, or 305 degrees F on a candy
- thermometer, about 7 minutes.
- Whisk the butter and salt into the sugar mixture.
- Gradually pour in the cream and vanilla taking care since the mixture
- will bubble up.

- Reduce the heat to medium and continue to cook, stirring
- occasionally, until the sugar reaches soft ball stage, 240 degrees F
- on the thermometer, about 5 minutes more.
- Immediately remove from the heat and cool for a minute.
- Ladle a couple tablespoons of warm caramel over some of the nut
- clusters, to make the spider bodies.
- Then press 6 pieces of licorice into the warm caramel to make the
- legs.
- Repeat with the remaining caramel and licorice.
- (It's helpful to have an extra hand here, since the caramel can set
- quickly.
- If caramel hardens, warm over very low heat.)
- Let spiders cool 15 minutes.
- ~
- Meanwhile, put the chocolates in a medium heatproof bowl.
- Bring a saucepan filled with 1-inch or so of water to a very slow
- simmer; set the bowl over, but not touching, the water.
- Stir the chocolate occasionally until melted and smooth.
- (Alternatively, put the chocolate in a medium microwave-safe bowl.
- Melt at 50 percent power in the microwave until soft, about 1 minute.
- Stir, and continue heat until completely melted, 2 to 3 minutes
- more.)
- ~
- Spoon about 1 tablespoon of melted chocolate on top of each spider.
- Sprinkle with jimmies or chocolate curls, if desired.
- Let cool until firm.

Direction

- Line 2 baking sheets with waxed paper and lightly spray with non-stick spray.
- Mound 30 small clusters of pecans, about 3 or 4 pecans each, spaced a couple inches apart on the pan.
- Make caramel: Warm the cream over low heat and keep warm while you cook the sugar.
- Put the sugar and corn syrup and in a deep, heavy-bottomed large saucepan.
- Cook over medium heat, stirring occasionally until the sugar dissolves.
- Stop stirring, raise heat to medium-high, and simmer until the sugar reaches the hard crack stage, or 305 degrees F on a candy thermometer, about 7 minutes.
- Whisk the butter and salt into the sugar mixture.
- Gradually pour in the cream and vanilla taking care since the mixture will bubble up.
- Reduce the heat to medium and continue to cook, stirring occasionally, until the sugar reaches soft ball stage, 240 degrees F on the thermometer, about 5 minutes more.
- Immediately remove from the heat and cool for a minute.
- Ladle a couple tablespoons of warm caramel over some of the nut clusters, to make the spider bodies.
- Then press 6 pieces of licorice into the warm caramel to make the legs.
- Repeat with the remaining caramel and licorice.
- (It's helpful to have an extra hand here, since the caramel can set quickly.
- If caramel hardens, warm over very low heat.)
- Let spiders cool 15 minutes.
- Meanwhile, put the chocolates in a medium heatproof bowl.
- Bring a saucepan filled with 1-inch or so of water to a very slow simmer; set the bowl over, but not touching, the water.
- Stir the chocolate occasionally until melted and smooth.
- (Alternatively, put the chocolate in a medium microwave-safe bowl.
- Melt at 50 percent power in the microwave until soft, about 1 minute.

- Stir, and continue heat until completely melted, 2 to 3 minutes more.)
- Spoon about 1 tablespoon of melted chocolate on top of each spider.
- Sprinkle with jimmies or chocolate curls, if desired.
- Let cool until firm.

142. Pecan Brittle Recipe

Serving: 8 | Prep: | Cook: 10mins | Ready in:

Ingredients

- 1 cup pecans
- 2 sticks butter
- 1 cup granulated sugar
- 1/4 cup water
- 1/8 teaspoon salt

Direction

- Sprinkle nuts on cookie sheet.
- Add all other ingredients in a medium saucepan.
- Cook over medium heat stirring constantly.
- When mixtures starts to turn caramel color pour over nuts.
- Allow to cool then break into pieces.

143. Pecan Clusters Recipe

Serving: 20 | Prep: | Cook: 8mins | Ready in:

Ingredients

- 1 jar marshmellow creme (7 oz)
- 1 1/2 pound milk chocolate kisses
- 5 cups sugar
- 1 can evaporated pet milk (13 oz)
- 2 cups butter
- 6 cups pecan halves

Direction

- Combine sugar, milk, and butter in saucepan; bring to a boil and cook 8 minutes, stirring constantly.
- Pour over marshmallow crème and kisses.
- Stir until well blended.
- Stir in pecans.
- Drop by teaspoonfuls onto wax paper.
- Makes about 12 dozen.

144. Pecan Diamonds From The Culinary Institute Of America Recipe

Serving: 48 | Prep: | Cook: 50mins | Ready in:

Ingredients

- cookie Dough
- 1 1/4 cups (2 1/2 sticks) unsalted butter, softened
- 3/4 cup sugar
- 1 whole egg
- 1 teaspoon vanilla extract
- 3 2/3 cups cake flour, sifted
- ....
- pecan Filling
- 2 cups (4 sticks) unsalted butter, cubed
- 2 cups light brown sugar, packed
- 1/2 cup sugar
- 1 cup honey
- 1/2 cup heavy cream
- 7 1/2 cups pecans, chopped

Direction

- Cookie Dough
- Cream together butter and sugar in a mixer bowl with the paddle attachment on medium speed until smooth and light, 1–2 minutes. Gradually incorporate egg and vanilla, stopping mixer and scraping bowl as necessary. Add flour and mix on low speed

until just blended, about 30 seconds. Do not overmix.
- Place dough onto parchment paper or a lightly floured surface and shape into a flat square. Wrap dough well with plastic wrap and refrigerate at least an hour.
- Preheat oven to 350 degrees F and line bottom of a 15-inch x 10-inch jelly roll pan with parchment.
- Roll dough out to a rectangle 17 inches x 12 inches x 1/8-inch thick. Transfer the rolled dough to the baking pan, gently pressing it to the pan. Trim the edges with a paring knife, and prick the bottom of the dough with the prongs of a fork to prevent bubbling during baking.
- Bake until dough is firm but has no color, about 10–12 minutes. Cool dough while you make the filling.
- ....
- Pecan Filling
- Place the butter, sugars, honey, and cream into a heavy-bottom saucepot. Bring mixture to a boil over medium-high heat and cook, stirring constantly, until it reaches 240 degrees F on a candy thermometer. Remove pot from the heat, add pecans, and stir until fully incorporated. Immediately pour into the pre-baked crust and spread into an even layer.
- Bake in 350 degree F oven until the filling bubbles evenly across the surface and the crust is golden brown, about 40 minutes. Cool thoroughly before cutting.
- Remove from pan using a knife to release the edges and invert the slab onto the back of a sheet pan. Transfer to a cutting board by flipping it over so it is right side up. Trim off the edges and cut into 1- or 2-inch diamonds.
- The bars store well at room temperature, but can also be refrigerated or frozen as long as wrapped airtight.

145. Pecan Divinity Recipe

Serving: 12 | Prep: | Cook: 15mins | Ready in:

Ingredients

- 1 1/2 cups sugar
- 1/2 cup light corn syrup (Karo brand preferred)
- 1/4 cup hot water
- 1/2 teaspoon white vinegar
- 1 stiffy beaten egg white
- 1/2 teaspoon vanilla
- 1/2 cup chopped pecans

Direction

- Combine the first four ingredients in a large saucepan, cover and place over medium heat until it boils. Cook to very hard ball stage (126 degrees) then remove from heat. Cool a bit then gradually add to stiff egg white. Beat constantly until very stiff. Let cool then add vanilla and nuts. Drop by spoonful on waxed paper and let set for an hour. Should stay very stiff and peaky if it turns out right but will be puddles if it doesn't. Still tastes good even if it doesn't set up stiff, but doesn't look very pretty.

146. Pecan Molasses Brittle Recipe

Serving: 810 | Prep: | Cook: 300mins | Ready in:

Ingredients

- 1 Cup sugar
- 1/2 Cup light corn syrup
- 1/2 Cup molasses
- 2 Cups whole pecans
- 1/2 Teaspoon salt
- 1 Teaspoon baking soda

Direction

- In a sauce pot combine the sugar, molasses, and corn syrup at medium-high heat. Stir and cook until the sugar dissolves (approximately 5 minutes).
- Add pecans and salt and cook another 12 minutes, stirring occasionally.
- After 12 minutes, quickly stir in your baking soda and then empty the contents into a greased cookie sheet (for this, I like to use the disposable cookie sheets because they are pliable and less of a chance of the brittle sticking to the cookie sheet).
- Place in the refrigerator for 5 hours or longer to harden.
- After 5 hours, remove from the refrigerator and with the end of a sturdy utensil crack, serve, and enjoy.

147. Pecan Penuche Recipe

Serving: 36 | Prep: | Cook: 40mins | Ready in:

Ingredients

- 1 cup packed light brown sugar
- 2 cups white sugar
- 1 cup milk
- 3 Tbsp. butter
- 1 teas. pure vanilla extract
- 1 cup pecans, coarsely chopped

Direction

- In a 3 quart saucepan combine the sugars and milk. Bring to a boil over medium heat, stirring constantly. Continue cooking without stirring until mixture reaches soft-ball stage (236 degrees F on a candy thermometer). Remove from heat. Add butter and vanilla - DO NOT STIR. Let the mixture cool until it reaches 110 degrees F. While the mixture is cooling, butter 8"X8" square pan. Line with foil so that it is overlapping by an inch or two on two ends. Butter foil.
- With a wooden spoon, beat mixture until it begins to lose its gloss. QUICKLY stir in pecans and pour into pan. DO NOT scrape the sides of the pot - they may be sugary. After mixture has cooled and set, lift out foil and cut penuche in 1 or 1-1/2 inch pieces.

148. Pecan Pralines Recipe

Serving: 5 | Prep: | Cook: 10mins | Ready in:

Ingredients

- 1 1/2 Tablespoons butter
- 16 ounce bag chopped pecans
- 1- Cup sugar
- 1 1/4- Cups brown sugar
- 6- Tablespoons water

Direction

- In medium saucepan combine sugar, water and butter.
- Turn burner to low heat, when mixture begins to boil rapidly, add the pecans.
- Continue to boil stirring constantly, until mixture forms large bubbles on top and has thickened.
- Remove from burner, then drop by teaspoonfuls onto well-buttered cookie sheet or wax paper.
- Let cool for two hours then serve.

149. Pecan Roll Recipe

Serving: 10 | Prep: | Cook: 10mins | Ready in:

Ingredients

- 1 cup cream
- 2 cups sugar
- 1/2 cup white corn syrup
- 1-1/2 cups pecans

- 1 cup light brown sugar

Direction

- Boil cream, sugar, syrup, to soft-ball stage. (234-238 F).
- Cool to room temperature then beat till creamy.
- Turn out onto board dusted with powdered sugar and knead until firm.
- Shape into a roll and cover the outside with pecans.
- Put in cool place to harden.
- Slice when firm with a sharp knife.

150. Pecan White Chocolate Brownies

Serving: 20 | Prep: | Cook: 20mins | Ready in:

Ingredients

- 2/3 Cups Butter (150g)
- 1 and 1/3 Cups White Chocolate (250g)
- 2 Large Eggs
- 2 tsp Vanilla Extract
- 1/3 Cup Brown Sugar (60g)
- 1 Cup Sugar (200g)
- 2 Cups All Purpose Flour (240g)
- 1/2 tsp Baking Soda
- 3/4 Cup Pecans, Chopped (95g)

Direction

- Preheat the oven to 180°C (350°F) and line an 9"x9" pan with baking paper.
- Melt the butter and white chocolate together.
- Beat the egg, brown sugar, sugar and vanilla extract together until light.
- Mix in the chocolate mixture.
- Mix in the flour, baking soda and chopped pecans.
- Bake for 25-35 minutes. The outside edges will be golden, the middle will sink slightly and the top will be crackly. The middle will also wobble slightly but this is a good as it will be nice and fudgy!
- Nutrition
- Serving: 1Piece | Calories: 260kcal | Carbohydrates: 36g | Protein: 3g | Fat: 12g | Saturated Fat: 7g | Cholesterol: 46mg | Sodium: 114mg | Potassium: 65mg | Fiber: 1g | Sugar: 24g | Vitamin A: 37IU | Vitamin C: 1mg | Calcium: 34mg | Iron: 1mg.

151. Pecan Chocolate Chip Cookie Brittle Recipe

Serving: 20 | Prep: | Cook: 19mins | Ready in:

Ingredients

- 1 1/2 cups all-purpose flour
- 1 tsp. baking powder
- 1/4 tsp. baking soda
- 1/4 tsp. salt
- 3/4 cup butter, melted and cooled slightly
- 1/2 cup granulated sugar
- 1/3 cup firmly packed light brown sugar
- 1 tsp. vanilla extract
- 1 cup semisweet chocolate mini-morsels
- 1 cup pecan pieces, toasted (see note)
- 1/2 cup sweetened flaked coconut, toasted (see note)

Direction

- Combine first 4 ingredients; set aside.
- Stir together butter and next 3 ingredients in a large bowl; add flour mixture, stirring until smooth. Stir in chocolate morsels, pecans, and coconut. (Dough will look crumbly.)
- Press dough evenly into a lightly greased 15" x 10" jelly-roll pan, pressing almost to edges.
- Bake at 350° for 19 minutes or until lightly browned and cookie "slab" seems crisp. Cool completely in pan. Break cookie into pieces.
- NOTE: You can toast pecan pieces and coconut in the same pan at 350° for 8 minutes.

152. Poor Mans Millionaires Recipe

Serving: 10 | Prep: | Cook: 15mins | Ready in:

Ingredients

- 1 pkg Carmels, (Kraft)
- 2 T canned milk
- 2 T margarine
- 3 C chopped pecans
- 1 large hershey bar
- Gulf paraffin wax

Direction

- In Double boiler melt caramels, milk and margarine, Add nuts and mix well.
- Drop spoonfuls onto waxed paper.
- Let candies cool.
- In Double boiler melt Hershey Bar with 1/3 bar of paraffin wax.
- Using a toothpick Dip Candy into chocolate, put onto waxed paper to cool.

153. Poppycock Recipe

Serving: 0 | Prep: | Cook: 1hours | Ready in:

Ingredients

- 6 c. popped corn
- 2 c. nuts (I use pecans)
- 1 1/3 c. brown sugar
- 1/2 c. corn syrup
- 1 c. margarine
- 1 t. vanilla

Direction

- 1. Pop your corn and let it cool completely.
- 2. Mix sugar, syrup and margarine on medium heat in a thick-bottomed saucepan.
- 3. Bubble this mixture for 25 minutes, stirring constantly.
- 4. Remove from the heat and add the vanilla.
- 5. Cool slightly.
- 6. Pour over the popcorn and nuts in large, lightly buttered glass or metal bowl and mix thoroughly with large, lightly buttered wooden or metal spoon.
- 7. Spread on lightly buttered cookie sheet(s) and leave overnight.
- 8. Store loosely in covered containers.
- Makes wonderful gifts.

154. Positively Yummy Pumpkin Fudge Recipe

Serving: 36 | Prep: | Cook: 35mins | Ready in:

Ingredients

- 3 cups white sugar
- 1 cup milk
- 3 Tablespoons light corn syrup
- 1/2 cup pumpkin puree
- 1/4 teaspoon salt
- 1 teaspoon pumpkin pie spice
- 1-1/2 teaspoons vanilla extract
- 1/2 cup butter
- 1/2 cup chopped walnuts/pecans (optional)

Direction

- Butter or grease one 8 x 8 inch pan.
- In a 3 quart saucepan, mix together sugar, milk, corn syrup, pumpkin and salt.
- Bring to a boil over high heat, stirring constantly.
- Reduce heat to medium and continue boiling.
- Do not stir.
- When mixture registers 232 degrees F (110 degrees C) on candy thermometer, or forms a soft ball when dropped into cold water, remove pan from heat.
- Stir in pumpkin pie spice, vanilla, butter and nuts.

- Cool to lukewarm (110 degrees F or 43 degrees C on candy thermometer).
- Beat mixture until it is very thick and loses some of its gloss.
- Quickly pour into a greased eight-inch pan.
- When firm cut into 36 squares.

155. Praline Grahams Recipe

Serving: 4 | Prep: | Cook: 12mins | Ready in:

Ingredients

- 12 graham crackers(4 3/4x 2 1/2in)
- 1/2C butter
- 1/2C packed brown sugar
- 1/2C finely chopped walnuts(pecans work well too)

Direction

- Line a 15"x10"x1" baking pan with heavy-duty foil
- Break graham crackers at indentations
- Place in a single layer in pan
- In a small saucepan, combine butter and brown sugar
- Bring to a rolling boil over medium heat
- Boil for 2 min
- Remove from heat
- Add nuts
- Pour over crackers
- Bake at 350 for 10 min or until lightly browned
- Let stand for 2-3 min
- Remove to a wire rack to cool

156. Praline Pecans Recipe

Serving: 8 | Prep: | Cook: 60mins | Ready in:

Ingredients

- 1 cup dark karo
- 1/2 cup sugar
- 1 lb. pecans (can use other nuts if desired)
- 2 tsp. water
- salt (as desired, on finished product)

Direction

- In a large skillet (I use a cast iron), combine Karo, sugar, and water.
- Cook on low heat until sugar dissolves.
- Put pecans into the karo mix and heat until the pecans become sticky/ tacky.
- Place the mixture of karo and nuts on to a large cookie sheet.
- Bake in the oven at 325° until the pecans are brown and the karo is bubbling.
- Pour onto foil to allow cooling.
- Sprinkle with salt.
- Break apart and store into ziploc bags. (Don't wait until they get hard to break apart. Try while they are still warm, but be cautious because they can burn your hands)

157. Pralines Anyone Recipe

Serving: 24 | Prep: | Cook: 15mins | Ready in:

Ingredients

- 1 Cup of light brown sugar, Firmly Packed
- 1 Cup of Garnulated sugar
- 1 Tbsp. light corn syrup
- 1 Tbsp. unsalted butter
- 5 Tbsp. of water
- 1 Cup Chopped pecans
- aluminum foil, Sprayed with nonstick cooking spray

Direction

- Combine the sugars, syrup, butter and 5 tbsps. of water in a sauce pan over medium heat. Bring to a boil. Add the pecans and continue cooking until the mixture reaches the soft ball stage. (238°F on the candy temp) remove the pan from the heat and stir vigorously with a wooden spoon until the candy begins to turn opaque. Quickly drop spoonful onto aluminum foil and allow to harden. Store the pralines in an air tight tin.

158. Pralines Recipe

Serving: 24 | Prep: | Cook: 20mins | Ready in:

Ingredients

- 4 cups brown sugar
- 2 cups heavy cream
- 2 tbs butter
- 1 tsp vanilla
- 2 cups pecans, chopped

Direction

- Butter a medium saucepan. It makes it easier to clean. Add cream and place on stove over high heat. Bring to boil and immediately add the sugar and stir rapidly until it dissolves. Stir in vanilla and pecans. Lower heat to medium and stir frequently. Bring to soft ball stage (236 on candy thermometer). Remove from heat and beat in butter. Candy will lose its gloss and become cloudy. On waxed paper, drop good size spoonful. Stir occasionally to keep ingredients combined. When pralines have cooled, remove. They will be hard to remove later.

159. Pralines With Pecans Recipe

Serving: 4 | Prep: | Cook: | Ready in:

Ingredients

- Pralines with pecans and evaporated milk, along with brown sugar, butter, and vanilla.

- Ingredients:
- •1 1/4 cups of sugar
- •3/4 cups of brown sugar
- •1/2 cup of evaporated milk
- •4 tablespoons butter
- •1 tablespoon vanilla
- •1 1/2 cups pecans

Direction

- Preparation:
- Put sugars & milk in heavy bottom pan & cook to soft ball stage. Take off fire & add frozen butter, vanilla & pecans & stir until shine leaves mixture & then spoon on waxed paper. Very easy & makes the best pralines ever.
- Candy - Making Chart
- Thread begins at 230° the syrup will make a 2" thread when dropped from a spoon.
- Soft Ball begins at 234° a small amount of syrup dropped into chilled water forms a ball, but flattens when picked up with fingers
- Firm Ball begins at 244° the ball will hold its shape and flatten only when pressed.
- Hard Ball begins at 250° the ball is more rigid but still pliable.
- Soft Crack begins at 270° when a small amount of syrup is dropped into chilled water it will separate into threads which will bend when picked up.
- Hard Crack begins at 300° the syrup separates into threads that are hard and brittle.
- Caramelized Sugar 310° to 338° between these temperatures the syrup will turn dark golden, but will turn black at 350°.

160. Pronto Pralines Recipe

Serving: 24 | Prep: | Cook: 78mins | Ready in:

Ingredients

- 1 4-serving size package regular (not instant!) vanilla pudding mix
- 1 cup packed browned sugar

- 1/2 cups sugar
- 1 5 ounce can evaporated milk
- 1 t vanilla
- 2 scant cups coarsely chopped pecans

Direction

- Step 1: Combine pudding mix, brown sugar, and sugar in a medium saucepan. Stir in evaporated milk. Bring mixture to a full boil, stirring constantly. Boil for 7-8 minutes, stirring occasionally.
- Step 2: Remove saucepan from heat; stir in vanilla. Beat three minutes; do not over beat. (Mixture should be shiny when dropped.) Stir in pecans.
- Step 3: Drop by tablespoon onto waxed paper. Let stand at room temperature 1 hour to harden. Makes 24.
- If you use a 6-serving pkg of pudding mix, increase all ingredients by 50%; make up the difference in evaporated milk with heavy cream if evap milk not available, increase boiling time to 8-9 minutes

161. Pumpkin Fudge Recipe

Serving: 16 | Prep: | Cook: 25mins | Ready in:

Ingredients

- 3 cups sugar
- 3/4 cup melted butter
- 2/3 cup evaporated milk
- 1/2 cup canned pumpkin
- 2 tablespoons corn syrup
- 1 teaspoon pumpkin pie spice
- 1 (12-ounce) package white chocolate morsels
- 1 (7-ounce) jar marshmallow crème
- 1 cup chopped pecans, toasted
- 1 teaspoon vanilla extract

Direction

- Line a 9x9 inch pan with aluminum foil, and set aside.
- Stir together first 6 ingredients in a 3 1/2-quart saucepan over medium-high heat, and cook, stirring constantly, until mixture comes to a boil. Cook, stirring constantly, until a candy thermometer registers 234° (soft-ball stage) or for about 12 minutes.
- Remove pan from heat; stir in remaining ingredients until well blended. Pour into a greased aluminum foil-lined 9-inch square pan. Let stand 2 hours or until completely cool; cut fudge into squares

162. Pumpkin Pie Fudge Recipe

Serving: 0 | Prep: | Cook: 30mins | Ready in:

Ingredients

- 2 cups granulated sugar
- 1 cup light brown sugar
- ¾ cup unsalted butter
- 2/3 cup or 5-ounce can evaporated milk
- ½ cup canned pumpkin
- 2 teaspoons pumpkin pie spice
- 2 cups white chocolate chips
- 1 (7 oz.) jar marshmallow creme
- 1 cup chopped pecans
- 1½ teaspoons vanilla extract

Direction

- Line a 9×13-inch baking pan with foil, leaving some hanging over the sides for easy removal.
- Combine the granulated sugar, brown sugar, evaporated milk, pumpkin, butter and spice in a medium saucepan.
- Bring to a full rolling boil over medium heat, stirring constantly.
- Boil, stirring constantly, for 10 to 12 minutes.
- Quickly stir in the white chocolate chips, marshmallow crème, pecans and vanilla extract.

- Stir vigorously for 1-2 minutes or until the chocolate chips are melted. Immediately pour into the prepared pan.
- Let stand on wire rack for 2 hours or until completely cooled. Refrigerate tightly covered overnight. Cut into 1 inch pieces.

163. Quick Nut Fudge Recipe

Serving: 0 | Prep: | Cook: 25mins | Ready in:

Ingredients

- 1 (16-ounce) package powdered sugar,
- sifted
- 1/2 cup cocoa
- 1/4 teaspoon salt
- 1/4 cup milk
- 1/4 cup plus 2 Tablespoons butter or
- margarine
- 1 Tablespoon vanilla extract
- 3/4 cup chopped pecans, divided

Direction

- Combine all ingredients except pecans in top of double boiler; bring water to a boil. Reduce heat and cook, stirring constantly, until mixture is smooth. Remove from heat; stir in 1/2 cup pecans.
- Quickly spread mixture into a lightly greased 9x5x3-inch loaf pan; sprinkle with remaining pecans. Chill until firm; cut into squares. Store in refrigerator.

164. ROLLO PRETZELS Recipe

Serving: 50 | Prep: | Cook: 23mins | Ready in:

Ingredients

- 50 small pretzel twists
- 50 pieces rollo candy
- 50 pieces whole pecans or walnuts

Direction

- Place pretzel pieces on a baking sheet.
- Top with one Rollo candy.
- Place in a warm oven (250 degrees) to just let the candy melt on top of the pretzel to hold it in place.
- Remove from oven and place a nut on top.
- Let cool and harden.

165. Raisin Cashew Chocolate Fudge Recipe

Serving: 15 | Prep: | Cook: 20mins | Ready in:

Ingredients

- 1 king size Hershey chocolate Bar.... (7 - 8 oz.)
- 12 oz. bag of Nestle's chocolate Dots --- mini semi sweet chocolate chips
- 1 cup cashews, unsalted, chopped
- 1/2 cup pecans ,chopped
- 1/2 -3/4 cup raisins
- 1 jar (7-8 oz.) marshmallow Fluff
- ....
- 1/3 cup butter
- 1 cup evaporated milk
- 4 1/2 cups superfine sugar
- extra butter

Direction

- In a large heavy bowl that can stand heat.
- Break up Hershey Bar into pieces.
- Add chocolate dots on top.
- Then add the nuts and then the raisins and top with marshmallow fluff.
- Put in a warm spot so the chocolate starts to soften.
- ....

- In a heavy pan, butter the sides and bottom of the pan heavily.
- Put in 1/3 cup of butter and the evaporated milk.
- Heat until warm.
- Slowly add the sugar. Stir after each addition.
- Make sure the dry sugar does not touch the sides of the pan.
- Don't stir too hard. You don't want the sugar mixture all over the sides of the pan.
- Heat slowly until the sugar is dissolved keep stirring.
- DON'T scrap the sides of the pan.
- Then turn the heat up to medium.
- Using a candy thermometer bring temperature to 230 - 232' F.
- Stir mixture to keep from burning.
- Pour hot sugar mixture over chocolate mixture in the bowl.
- DO NOT scrape the pot out.
- Use a new spoon and blend the together as quickly as possible.
- DON"T over mix. There will be some streaks of the fluff that's ok.
- Spread mixture on a well-buttered jelly roll pan. (Large spatula works).
- Work quickly. This fudge sets up very fast.
- Cover tightly with plastic wrap and then foil.
- Put in a cold spot for 4 hours. Cut into pieces.
- ………………………………………
- Keep wrapped tightly. This fudge dries out very fast.

166. Red Pepper Fudge Recipe

Serving: 10 | Prep: | Cook: 30mins | Ready in:

Ingredients

- 1C chopped pecans
- 1/2 stick salted butter
- 1/2 t ground red pepper
- 1+T natural sugar
- 1C Hersey's cocoa
- 2C natural sugar
- 2 C 2% All Natural milk
- 2t vanilla
- 4T melted sweet butter

Direction

- Ok this is the way we did it, in a small pot I start the pecans.
- 1C chopped pecans
- ½ stick sated butter
- Cook these until they start getting a slight roasted taste then add
- 1/2t ground red pepper (New Mexico red/pizza pepper)
- 1T heaping Florida Crystals all natural sugar
- Cook this until the sugar starts to caramelize.
- Add this to the fudge when it (fudge) gets to around 200 deg and cook according to fudge recipe. I had to redo mine because we didn't take it to 240 deg. First time, the thermometer was touching the bottom of the pot.
- This is the recipe used.
- 2C natural sugar
- 1C Hershey's cocoa
- 2C 2% promise land milk
- 2t real vanilla
- 4T melted sweet butter
- Combine these ingredients in a 3-4qt pot and cook for a bit and when around 200 add the pecan mix. Continue until the thermometer goes to the "soft ball" stage then cool it stirring like a mad man until thickening begins. Pour on/in a greased pan let it rest (I let mine set till next day)
- Watch it. It wants to stick while going for 230-240.

167. Reindeer Nibbles Recipe

Serving: 10 | Prep: | Cook: | Ready in:

Ingredients

- 1 large bag M & M candy pieces
- 1 can peanuts (any Variety)
- 3/4 cup raisins
- 3/4 cup or 1 package dry pineapple
- 1 pkg peanut butter/chocolate chips (6 oz size)
- 1 large can chow mein noodles
- 1 cup pecan pieces
- 3/4 cup craisins (dry cranberries)
- 3/4 cup almond slices

Direction

- Mix all ingredients together and store in a large zip top bag.
- Package and share.
- Use your own imagination and you can add or substitute on some of these ingredients.

168. Rich Creamy Pistachio Tangerine Fudge Recipe

Serving: 64 | Prep: | Cook: 10mins | Ready in:

Ingredients

- 1 11.5-ounce package milk chocolate pieces
- 1 14-ounce can sweetened condensed milk
- 8 ounces bittersweet or semisweet chocolate, coarsely chopped
- 2 to 3 teaspoons finely shredded tangerine or orange peel
- 1 teaspoon vanilla
- 1/2 cup chopped pistachios, toasted almonds or toasted pecans
- 1/2 cup white baking pieces
- Coarsely chopped pistachios, toasted almonds or toasted pecans (optional)

Direction

- Line an 8x8x2-inch or 9x9x2-inch baking pan with foil, extending the foil over the edges of the pan. Butter the foil; set pan aside.
- In a 2-quart heavy saucepan, combine milk chocolate pieces, condensed milk, and bittersweet or semisweet chocolate. Cook and stir over low heat until chocolate just melts and mixture is well combined and smooth. Remove saucepan from heat. Stir in tangerine or orange peel and vanilla.
- Immediately spread half of fudge into the prepared pan; sprinkle with pistachios and white baking pieces; press in lightly. Spread remaining fudge evenly on top. If you like, sprinkle with additional nuts; press in lightly. Score into squares while warm. Cover and chill at least 2 hours or until firm. When fudge is firm, use foil to lift fudge out of pan. Cut fudge into 1-inch squares. Store tightly covered in the refrigerator for up to 1 month.
- Makes about 2-1/2 pounds (64 pieces).
- Recipe Note: This candy recipe directs you to line your pan with foil. But how do you get that foil pushed into those corners without tearing it? Try this: Shape the foil around the outside of your pan, then lift it off and place it inside the pan, pressing gently into the corners.

169. Rocky Road Balls Recipe

Serving: 30 | Prep: | Cook: 10mins | Ready in:

Ingredients

- 5 oz miniature marshmellows
- 1 1/2 finely chopped pecans
- 5 oz regular raisins
- 1 1/4 cup peanut butter
- 2 tbsp powder sugar
- 1 pkg chocolate almond bark (melting chocolate)
- 1-1 1/2 cup powdered sugar (dusting hands and rolling mixture balls in)

Direction

- Melt almond bark on double boiler. Until all melted.

- In the meantime, in a large bowl, mix marshmallows, pecans, raisins, peanut butter & 2 tbsp. powdered sugar together, thoroughly. Mixture will be stiff but gooey. Make sure all in combined, takes a few minutes but will bind.
- Take 1-1 1/2 cups of powdered sugar place in a shallow bowl. Dust hands with powdered sugar, and grab about 1 1/2- 2 tbsp. of the mixture, it's an eyeball thing, roll in powdered sugar and in hand to make the lumpy balls (excuse the phase, I see how I worded it-- sorry) place on a parchment lined cookie sheet, Repeat dusting hands and rolling each lumpy ball until mixture is all gone. Let balls rest for a couple minutes before dipping into melted chocolate.
- Dip each ball quickly in melted chocolate. Shake off excess chocolate as best as you can. Place back on parchment lined pan. You may have extra chocolate, and mixture makes roughly 30 to 40 or so balls. Let balls cool completely until set and chocolate easily releases from the parchment.

170. Rocky Road Fudge Recipe

Serving: 24 | Prep: | Cook: 10mins | Ready in:

Ingredients

- 1 c. butterscotch (or mint) chips
- 1 c. chocolate chips (I used 60% cacao, but semi-sweet is fine)
- 14 oz condensed milk
- 2 c. nuts (walnuts, pecans or peanuts, optional)
- 2 c. marshmallows.

Direction

- Melt the chips together.
- Stir in Condensed Milk.
- Add nuts.

- Stir in marshmallows, don't stir too much or they will melt!
- Pour into a greased or lined 9x9" pan.
- Cool, slice, enjoy!

171. Rolo Pretzel Turtles Recipe

Serving: 48 | Prep: | Cook: 3mins | Ready in:

Ingredients

- 48 Rolo candies, unwrapped (Rolos are small round caramels dipped in chocolate)
- 48 pretzel rings
- 48 whole pecans

Direction

- No need to grease the cookie sheet – just lay the pretzel rings out on it, and place a Rolo candy on top of each ring.
- Bake at 350 degrees for 3 minutes (no more or you will have a melted mess!).
- Remove pan from oven and immediately place a whole pecan on each Rolo and gently push it down just a bit.
- Allow the candies to cool on the cookie sheet, letting the chocolate harden back up again before removing them to a storage container.

172. Rose Water And Ginger Poached Pears With Caramel Glaze On A Bed Of Crunch Vanilla Cream Recipe

Serving: 4 | Prep: | Cook: 1mins | Ready in:

Ingredients

- Poached pears
- 4 pears

- 500 ml of rose water
- A large piece of ginger
- vanilla cream
- 250 g of marscopone
- 50 g of chopped pecans
- 1 vanilla pod
- 1 tablespoon of vanilla essence
- 1 tablespoons of lemon juice
- caramel glaze
- 200ml water
- 4 tablespoons of brown sugar.
- 200ml of orange juice
- 1 stick of butter

Direction

- For the vanilla cream.
- Take vanilla from pod.
- In a non-stick pan toast pecans no oil or butter necessary.
- In a bowl put the mascarpone, vanilla, vanilla essence, toasted pecans and lemon juice.
- Beat with an electric whisk for 5 minutes.
- Chill for an hour.
- For the pears.
- De core the pears.
- Pour the rose water and put the ginger chunk into the saucepan.
- Bring to the boil.
- Put the pears into the saucepan and cover with a lid
- Let simmer for 20 minutes.
- When finished take out and let cool.
- For the caramel glaze.
- Put the butter and sugar into a saucepan and melt.
- Then pour in the water and orange juice and stir.
- To serve
- Spoon vanilla cream onto 4 plates.
- Place a pear on top of each bed.
- Pour caramel over the top.

173. Rum Balls Recipe

Serving: 0 | Prep: | Cook: |Ready in:

Ingredients

- 1/2 cups (140 grams) toasted pecans, finely chopped (hazelnuts, walnuts, or almonds can be used)
- 1 1/4 cups (120 grams) finely crushed vanilla wafer cookies or shortbread cookies
- 1/2 cup (55 grams) confectioners sugar (powdered or icing)
- 2 tablespoons (12 grams) cocoa powder (can used Dutch processed or regular unsweetened cocoa powder)
- 2 tablespoons light corn syrup
- 1/4 cup (60 ml) rum
- Garnish:
- 1/2 cup (55 grams) confectioners sugar (powdered or icing), sifted

Direction

- Toast nuts: Preheat oven to 350 degrees F (177 degrees C) and have rack in center of oven. Place the pecans on a baking sheet and toast for about 8 minutes, or until lightly browned and fragrant. Let cool completely and then either chop up finely with a knife or place in your food processor and pulse until finely chopped. Transfer to a large bowl.
- Process the vanilla wafer cookies or shortbread cookies in the food processor until finely ground. Add the crumbs to the finely chopped pecans. To this mixture add the confectioners' sugar and cocoa powder and stir until combined. Add the corn syrup and rum and mix well. Chill if necessary and then shape into 1 inch (2.5 cm) balls. Place the sifted confectioners' sugar into a small bowl and roll the rum balls in the sugar.
- Store in an airtight container in the refrigerator. These are best if made several days in advance of serving to allow the flavors to mingle.
- Serve at room temperature.
- Makes about 4 dozen (48 rum balls).

174. Rum Raisin Fudge Recipe

Serving: 0 | Prep: | Cook: 2hours | Ready in:

Ingredients

- 1 C. Raisins
- 1/2 C. Dark Rum
- 2 1/2 C. Granulated Sugar
- 1 C. Evaporated Milk
- 1/2 C. butter or Margarine
- 2 C. Dark chocolate chips
- 1 Jar (7 oz.) Marshmallow Creme
- 1/2 C. Chopped Pecans
- 1 T. Rum Extract

Direction

- In a small bowl combine raisins and rum. Cover and marinate overnight at room temperature.
- In a heavy large saucepan combine sugar, evaporated milk, and butter. Cook over medium heat stirring constantly, until mixture reaches soft ball stage (238 degrees on a candy thermometer).
- Remove from heat.
- Stir in chocolate chips, marshmallow crème, pecans, rum extract and raisin mixture.
- Spread mixture into a lightly greased 10 x 8 x 2" baking pan. Cool and cut into squares.

175. SOUTHERN PRALINES Recipe

Serving: 212 | Prep: | Cook: 20mins | Ready in:

Ingredients

- 2 CUPS sugar
- 3/4 TSP SODA
- 1 TSP butter
- 1 CUP light cream
- 2 CUPS pecan halves

Direction

- Combine sugar and soda in 3-quart saucepans
- Mix well
- Stir in cream
- Bring to boil over medium heat, stirring constantly
- Cook and stir to soft ball stage (234 degrees)
- Mixture caramelizes slightly as it cooks
- Remove from heat
- Add butter
- Stir in pecans
- Beat until thick enough to drop from spoon (takes 2 to 3 minutes)
- Drop from tablespoon onto waxed paper
- If candy becomes too stiff, add a tablespoon hot water
- Makes 2 1/2 dozen

176. SPIRIT BALLS Recipe

Serving: 20 | Prep: | Cook: | Ready in:

Ingredients

- 2 (7 oz.) pkg. pitted dates
- 1 c. pecans
- 1 ½ c. vanilla wafer crumbs
- ¼ c. sugar
- ¼ c. brandy or rum
- 2 tbsp. corn syrup
- coconut, flake or short cut or bakers dry chocolate powder.

Direction

- Put dates and nuts through food chopper.
- Crush wafers into fine crumbs.

- Mix all ingredients, except coconut, together; roll into ½ inch balls. Roll in coconut or chocolate.
- Place in tightly covered container.
- Let season for a few days.
- Yields 6 dozen.
- You can replace the "Spirits" with apple juice and just add a 1/4 teaspoon of brandy or rum flavoring.

177. Saltine Toffee Cookies Recipe

Serving: 12 | Prep: | Cook: 5mins | Ready in:

Ingredients

- * 4 ounces saltine crackers
- * 1 cup butter
- * 1 cup dark brown sugar
- * 2 cups semisweet chocolate chips
- * 3/4 cup chopped pecans

Direction

- Preheat oven to 400 degrees F (205 degrees C).
- Line cookie sheet with saltine crackers in single layer.
- In a saucepan combine the sugar and the butter. Bring to a boil and boil for 3 minutes. Immediately pour over saltines and spread to cover crackers completely.
- Bake at 400 degrees F (205 degrees C) for 5 to 6 minutes. Remove from oven and sprinkle chocolate chips over the top. Let sit for 5 minutes. Spread melted chocolate and top with chopped nuts. Cool completely and break into pieces.

178. Salty Chocolate Pecan Candy Recipe

Serving: 134 | Prep: | Cook: 15mins | Ready in:

Ingredients

- 1 cup pecans, coarsely chopped
- 3 (4-oz.) bars bittersweet chocolate baking bars
- 3 (4-oz.) white chocolate baking bars
- 1 teaspoon coarse sea salt*

Direction

- Place pecans in a single layer on a baking sheet.
- Bake at 350° for 8 to 10 minutes or until toasted.
- Line a 17- x 12-inch jelly-roll pan with parchment paper.
- Break each chocolate bar into 8 equal pieces. (You will have 48 pieces total.)
- Arrange in a checkerboard pattern in jelly-roll pan, alternating white and dark chocolate. (Pieces will touch.)
- Bake at 225° for 5 minutes or just until chocolate is melted.
- Remove pan to a wire rack.
- Swirl chocolates into a marble pattern using a wooden pick. Sprinkle evenly with toasted pecans and salt.
- Chill 1 hour or until firm. Break into pieces.
- Store in an airtight container in refrigerator up to 1 month.
- *3/4 tsp. kosher salt may be substituted.
- Note: For testing purposes only, we used Ghirardelli 60% Cacao Bittersweet Chocolate Baking Bars and Ghirardelli White Chocolate Baking Bars.

179. Salty Sweet Treat Recipe

Serving: 10 | Prep: | Cook: 2mins | Ready in:

Ingredients

- 20 mini pretzels
- 20 rolo candy pieces (I could not find the regular size ones so bought a bag of Minis and used 2 per pretzel)
- assorted "deluxe" nut mix, salted (cashews, pecans, brazil nuts and almonds are great)

Direction

- Lay pretzels on cookie sheet.
- Place rolos on top.
- Put in oven at 350 for only a few minutes - so rolos are very soft but still have their shape.
- Take them out of oven and quickly smoosh a nut down on each pretzel.
- Cool the tray in the fridge for about 15 minutes.
- Carefully remove them from the tray (may need a spatula).
- Serve cold or at room temperature.

180. Seaside Candy Rolls Recipe

Serving: 24 | Prep: | Cook: | Ready in:

Ingredients

- 2 cups pecans, divided
- 1/3 cup margarine or butter
- 1/3 cup light corn syrup
- 1 tsp. maple flavoring
- 1/2 tsp. salt
- 1 box (1 lb.) powdered sugar, sifted
- corn syrup for brushing rolls

Direction

- Chop 3/4 cups nuts finely and 1-1/4 cups nuts coarsely. Set aside. Mix butter, corn syrup, flavoring and salt. Add sugar all at once and knead with hands until smooth. (It takes a while so be patient!) Knead in the fine nuts. Divide dough into two. Roll each into 2 inch wide logs. Brush with corn syrup roll in coarse nuts. Wrap in wax paper, chill until firm. Slice into 1/4 inch pieces.
- Makes 1-1/2 pounds
- *Note this is what I do and it makes less of a mess. I divide the coarse nuts amongst two pieces of waxed paper. Place each log onto the nut covered wax paper. Brush log with corn syrup turning until most of the log is covered in the nuts. Then just roll up pressing the paper and nuts around the log. Less mess!

181. Sees Fudge The Best Recipe

Serving: 20 | Prep: | Cook: 8mins | Ready in:

Ingredients

- 18 ounces of semi-sweet or bittersweet chocolate chips (1 1/2 bags)
- 3 cups chopped walnuts or pecans
- (I have used "cocktail-style" peanuts and its good if you want a peanut flavor.)
- 1 cup of regular butter (2 sticks) Do not use margarine!
- 1 can (13 ounces) evaporated milk
- 4 cups of mini marshmallows or 20 large marshmallows, cut up
- 4 cups granulated sugar (no substitutes!)
- 2 teas. vanilla extract
- **All of your ingredients should be a room temperature!

Direction

- Put your marshmallows, chips, butter and vanilla in a large bowl.
- In a heavy pot, add the sugar and milk and bring to a boil over a medium flame.
- Bring this to a rolling boil and cook for exactly eight (8) minutes

- Pour the milk and sugar over the marshmallows, chips, butter and vanilla and let it all sit for a minute.
- Start stirring with a wooden spoon until the marshmallows have melted and add the nuts and stir until the fudge is smooth.
- Pour into a 9x13 pan or a 15x13 sheet pan. (I use a 9x13 disposable aluminium pan.)
- Cover your pan with aluminum foil. (You do not have to butter your pan before pouring your fudge into it.)
- Let fudge rest and cure overnight or for at least several hours until firm to the touch.
- *You can add more or less nuts as per your preference.
- *I have added items like M&M's during the holidays, pretzel pieces, used cashews (which was interesting!), toasted coconut, and even bits of vanilla wafers. The fudge without the nuts is excellent as well! You can even roll it into small balls and then roll it in chopped nuts for Fudge Truffles. You can add more mini-marshmallows AFTER you've mixed the fudge together for a Rocky Road Fudge.
- *This fudge is very soft before it sets as is MOST fudge. After you mix it that you can use a character cake pan and fill that with the fudge but if you do, spray the pan first with an anti-stick spray of some kind. (Bunny-shaped fudge for Easter, Santa-shaped or Xmas tree-shaped fudge)
- ___*You can always put the fudge in the fridge if you find that it hasn't set firmly enough to slice.
- *You can pour this into several small aluminum loaf pans for gift baskets or in round decorated tins for the holidays.
- **See's Candy is now $15.00 a pound!
- Serving suggestion: This fudge is best when served at room temperature.

182. Simple Yummies Recipe

Serving: 24 | Prep: | Cook: 5mins | Ready in:

Ingredients

- 24 Rolo candies
- 24 pretzel Snaps
- 24 pecan halves

Direction

- Preheat oven to 350.
- Unwrap the Rolos.
- Place the Snaps on a parchment lined cookie sheet.
- Top with one Rolo each.
- Place in the oven for 4 minutes - yes, four!
- Take the sheet out and while still warm, press the Pecans into the candy.
- Let cool and serve.

183. Some Kinda Rich Fudge Dated 1964 Recipe

Serving: 16 | Prep: | Cook: 20mins | Ready in:

Ingredients

- 1/2 stick unsalted butter
- 12 ounces semisweet chocolate chips
- 12 ounces milk chocolate chips
- 1 teaspoon vanilla extract
- 1 teaspoon imitation butter flavor
- 14 ounces marshmallow crème
- 2 cups pecans chopped
- 1 large can evaporated milk
- 4-1/2 cups granulated sugar

Direction

- Line cookie sheet with aluminum foil then butter foil and set aside.
- Place chips, flavors, half the marshmallow crème and nuts in large saucepan.
- In separate saucepan bring milk and sugar to rolling boil while stirring constantly.
- Add butter and marshmallow crème.

- Bring back to a rolling boil and continue to boil 8 minutes.
- Remove from heat and pour mixture over chips, vanilla and nuts without scraping sides.
- Mix thoroughly and pour into prepared pan then cool 3 hours at room temperature.
- Remove from pan then remove foil and cut into squares.

184. Spiced Nuts Recipe

Serving: 16 | Prep: | Cook: 45mins | Ready in:

Ingredients

- 1 lb nuts (pecans or walnuts, halves or large pieces are best)
- 2 egg whites
- 1 tbsp water
- 1 cup sugar
- 1 tsp cinnamon
- 1 tsp salt

Direction

- Preheat oven to 300oF.
- Mix together egg whites and water and whisk until foamy.
- Stir in nuts.
- Add sugar, cinnamon, and salt.
- Stir well to coat and evenly mix.
- Pour onto a baking sheet (line it with foil or a silicone) and place in oven.
- Stir nuts thoroughly every 15 minutes for a total of 45 minutes.
- Remove from oven and cool.

185. Spiced Pumpkin Fudge Recipe

Serving: 48 | Prep: | Cook: 15mins | Ready in:

Ingredients

- 2cups granulated sugar
- 1 cup packed light borwn sugar
- 1 1/2 sticks of butter
- 2/3 cup evaporated milk
- 1/2 cup pumpkin
- 2 teaspoon pumpkin pie spice
- 2 cups white morsels (12 oz)
- 1 (7oz) marshmallow creme
- 1 cup chopped pecans
- 1 1/2 t. vanilla

Direction

- Line an oblong cake pan with foil.
- Combine sugar, brown sugar, evaporated milk, pumpkin, butter and spice in medium, heavy duty saucepan.
- Bring to a full rolling boil over medium heat, stirring constantly for 10 to 12 minutes or until candy thermometer reaches 234 degrees to 240 degrees, the soft ball stage.
- Quickly stir in morsels, crème, nuts and vanilla.
- Stir vigorously for 1 minute or until morsels are melted.
- Immediately pour into prepared pan.
- Stand on wire rack for two hours or until completely cool.
- Refrigerate tightly covered.
- To cut, lift from pan and remove foil.
- Makes 48 2" pieces.

186. Sugar Cookie Chocolate Crunch Fudge Recipe

Serving: 48 | Prep: | Cook: 10mins | Ready in:

Ingredients

- 2 tablespoons light corn syrup
- 2 tablespoons butter or margarine
- 1/4 teaspoon salt

- 1 can (14 oz) sweetened condensed milk (not evaporated)
- 1 roll (16.5 oz) Create 'n Bake refrigerated sugar cookies, cut into small chunks
- 2 bags (12 oz each) semisweet chocolate chips
- 5 teaspoons vanilla
- 6 pecan crunch crunchy granola bars (3 pouches from 8.9-oz box), coarsely crushed (heaping 1 cup)*
- Fresh mint sprigs, if desired

Direction

- In 3-quart heavy saucepan or deep 10-inch non-stick skillet, cook corn syrup, butter, salt and condensed milk over medium heat 2 to 3 minutes, stirring constantly with wooden spoon, until well blended. Reduce heat to medium-low; stir in cookie dough chunks. Cook 3 to 5 minutes, stirring constantly, until mixture is smooth and candy thermometer reads 160°F. Remove from heat.
- Stir in chocolate chips and vanilla until chips are melted and mixture is smooth. Add crushed granola bars; stir until well blended. Cook over low heat 1 to 2 minutes, stirring constantly, until mixture is shiny. Spread in ungreased 12x8-inch or 13x9-inch pan.** Refrigerate uncovered at least 2 hours or until firm.
- Cut into 8 rows by 6 rows. Serve in decorative candy cups or mini paper baking cups on platter garnished with mint sprigs.

187. Sugar Free Chocolate Fudge Recipe

Serving: 16 | Prep: | Cook: 480mins | Ready in:

Ingredients

- Ngredients:
- 2 packages (8-oz each) 1/3 less fat cream cheese
- 2 Squares (1-oz each) unsweetened chocolate, melted and cooled
- 24 packets sugar substitute (equivalent to ½ cup sugar or using stevia (a natural herb sugar substitute), you use less than regular sugar subs ... 2 tbsp is equal in flavor for 1/2 cup .
- stevia is relatively expensive to buy, but it lasts a long time!
- 1 tsp. vanilla extract
- ½ cup chopped pecans

Direction

- In a small mixing bowl, beat the cream cheese, chocolate, sweetener and vanilla until smooth. Stir in pecans. Pour into an 8-inch square baking pan lined with foil. Cover and refrigerate overnight. Cut into 16 squares. Serve chilled.
- Serving size 1 piece
- Nutrition Values: Calories per serving: 147, Sodium: 84mg, Fat: 14gm, Cholesterol: 31mg, Carbohydrate: 5gm, Protein: 3gm
- Diabetic Exchanges: 3 fat
- Note: This recipe is Diabetic Friendly, Gastric Bypass Friendly, and anyone can eat this.

188. Sugared Nuts Delight Recipe

Serving: 1 | Prep: | Cook: 45mins | Ready in:

Ingredients

- * 1 egg white
- * 1/2 teaspoon water
- * 1/2 cup sugar
- * 1/2 teaspoon salt
- * 3/4 teaspoon cinnamon
- * 1/2 pound raw nuts such as: pecans or walnuts

Direction

- Preheat oven to 300 degrees F. Beat (with fork) egg white and water in large bowl. Combine sugar, salt, cinnamon on resealable bag. Shake. Place nuts in egg mixture. Drain back into bowl with slotted spoon.
- Shake in bag. Spread out in foil-lined pan. Bake for 30 to 45 minutes.
- If doubling, do one half at a time, but bake all at once.

189. Swedish Candied Nuts Recipe

Serving: 8 | Prep: | Cook: 40mins | Ready in:

Ingredients

- 1/2 pound (1 1/2 cups) almonds, blanched
- 1/2 pound (2 cups) pecan halves (original had walnuts)
- 1 cup sugar
- 1 tsp cinnamon (not in original)
- 1//2 tsp vanilla extract (not in original)
- dash salt
- 2 stiff-beaten egg whites
- 1/2 cup butter

Direction

- Preheat oven to 325 F.
- Toast nuts in oven till light brown. Stir a few times. Takes about 10 minutes. Let cool while preparing the rest.
- Fold sugar, cinnamon, vanilla, and salt into egg whites. Beat till stiff peaks form. Fold nuts into meringue.
- Melt butter in a jelly roll pan (15.5x10.5x1"). Spread nut mixture over butter.
- Bake in 325 F oven for about 30 minutes. Stir every 10 minutes, or till nuts are coated with a brown covering and no butter remains in bottom of pan.
- Tip onto foil. Cool. Break apart chunks. Store in jar or tin.
- Makes about 4 cups

190. Sweet Autumn Spiced Pecans Recipe

Serving: 5 | Prep: | Cook: 30mins | Ready in:

Ingredients

- 1 egg white
- 2 TB water
- 1/2 cup sugar
- 1/4 tsp allspice (I used pumpkin pie spice, works fine too)
- 1/4 tsp cloves
- 1/2 tsp cinnamon
- 1/2 tsp salt
- 2 1/2 cups pecans (large pieces or halves best for this recipe)

Direction

- Preheat oven to 300 degrees.
- Beat egg white and water until foamy (but not to soft peak).
- Add sugar, spices and salt and let stand until sugar dissolves (about 15 mins).
- Stir in nuts and mix well, coating all pieces.
- Spread mixture on large foil-lined baking sheet.
- Bake for 25-45 mins (depends on your oven), stirring every 15 mins.
- Remove from oven before too brown, mixture will still be foamy, let sit until hard (10-15 mins) and break apart.
- Put in bowl and watch them disappear!
- P.S. I also sprinkled them with some finely shredded bittersweet baking chocolate when I removed them from the oven, just cause I LOVE chocolate.

191. Sweet Spiced Fancy Nuts Recipe

Serving: 112 | Prep: | Cook: 20mins | Ready in:

Ingredients

- 1 egg white
- 1 tsp water
- 1 tsp vanilla
- 5 cups whole or halved nuts (pecans, almonds, walnuts, etc)
- 1/4 cup butter
- 1 cup sugar
- 1 tsp ground cinnamon
- 1/4 tsp ground nutmeg
- 1/4 tsp ground allspice
- 1/2 tsp salt

Direction

- Preheat oven 325 F.
- Melt butter in a15x10x1-inch baking pan (jelly roll/bar pan).
- In large mixing bowl, beat egg white and water till soft peaks form. Add vanilla beat a bit longer.
- Fold in nuts until thoroughly coated.
- Combine sugar, cinnamon, nutmeg, allspice, and salt. Sprinkle over nut mixture.
- Toss until nuts are thoroughly coated.
- Spread nuts in prepared pan. Bake at 325F for 20 minutes. Stir after 10 minutes to ensure even browning.
- When done, turn out onto foil or wax paper. Cool. Break chunks into smaller pieces. Store in airtight container.

192. Sweet Swedish Pecans Recipe

Serving: 12 | Prep: | Cook: 40mins | Ready in:

Ingredients

- 1 pound good quality, large pecans
- 2 stiffly beaten egg whites
- 1 cup sugar
- dash of salt
- ½ cup butter

Direction

- Spread pecans out on a large cookie sheet and toast them at 350 degrees until browned just a bit.
- Remove pan from oven and cool nuts completely.
- Reduce oven temperature to 325 degrees.
- Beat egg whites until stiff peaks form.
- Slowly add sugar and salt, and beat just to blend.
- Add cooled nuts and stir gently until all are coated.
- Place butter on a heavy duty cookie sheet; put pan in oven until butter is completely melted.
- Remove pan from oven and spread coated nuts in the butter, keeping them in a single layer.
- Bake for 30 minutes, stirring every 10 minutes, until nuts are covered with a light brown coating.
- Cool and store in covered container.

193. THREE CHOCOLATE FUDGE WITH PECANS Recipe

Serving: 48 | Prep: | Cook: 15mins | Ready in:

Ingredients

- Ingredients:
- 3 1/3 cups sugar
- 1 cup butter or margarine
- 1 cup packed dark sugar
- 1 can (12-oz) evaporated milk
- 32 large marshmallows, halved
- 2 cups (12-oz) semisweet chocolate chips

- 2 milk chocolate candy bars (7-oz each) broken
- 2 squares (1-oz each) semisweet baking chocolate, chopped
- 1 tsp. vanilla extract
- 2 cups chopped pecans

Direction

- In a large saucepan, combine first four ingredients. Cook and stir over medium heat until sugar is dissolved. Bring to a rapid boil; boil for 5 minutes, stirring constantly. Remove from the heat; stir in marshmallows until melted. Stir in chocolate chips until melted. Add chocolate bars and baking chocolate; stir until melted. Fold in vanilla and pecans; mix well. Pour into a greased 15-inch x 10-inch x 1-inch baking pan. Chill until firm. Cut into squares.

194. Texas Millionaire Candy Recipe

Serving: 12 | Prep: | Cook: 5mins | Ready in:

Ingredients

- 8 oz of caramels
- 2 Tablespoons milk
- 2 Cups Chopped Texas pecans
- 8 oz of The Best chocolate you can afford
- Small amount of Paraffin

Direction

- In saucepan, melt caramels with the milk.
- Stir in the pecans.
- Drop by spoonful onto a waxed lined cookie sheet, chill.
- In another saucepan, melt the chocolate and paraffin.
- Roll the caramel, nut portions in the melted chocolate, place onto cookie sheet and chill.

195. Texas Style Microwave Pralines Recipe

Serving: 12 | Prep: | Cook: 13mins | Ready in:

Ingredients

- 1 cup whip cream
- 1 box dark brown sugar
- 2 Tablespoons margarine or butter
- 2 cups pecan pieces (not broken too small)
- chocolate chips (optional)

Direction

- Stir together whip cream and dark brown sugar in very large microwave safe mixing bowl. Zap in microwave on high for 13 minutes. Open microwave about half way through cooking time and give the mixture a stir or two to make sure it is mixed well. When time is up, take bowl out of microwave, add butter and stir until butter is melted. Add nuts, stir for a couple of minutes or so until mixture starts to thicken slightly. Quickly drop by spoonfuls on a sheet of foil. Allow pralines to cool and then put them in a covered container. If mixture is removed from bowl too quickly (too hot and shiny), the pralines will be too thin and may remain sticky. If the first one spreads out too much just put it back in the bowl and stir mixture for a minute or so more. If mixture gets to cool (dull in appearance) before it is spooned out on foil, it may become too firm to make individual pralines, but it can always be broken into chunks and eaten. Less attractive, but still good. Make a couple of batches and you will be able to tell when the mixture is right for spooning. Chocolate lovers can add 1/2 cup of chocolate chips to hot mixture along with the butter. The chips will melt completely producing "chocolate pralines".

196. The Best Christmas Fudge Recipe

Serving: 70 | Prep: | Cook: 10mins | Ready in:

Ingredients

- 1 cup milk
- 2 sticks unsalted butter
- 4 cups sugar
- 25 large marshmallows
- 12 ounces semi-sweet chocolate chips
- 2 ounces unsweetened chocolate
- 13 ounces big Hershey Bars
- 1 tablespoon pure vanilla extract
- 1 cup hand chopped pecans

Direction

- In heavy Dutch oven, heat milk, butter, and sugar until melted and dissolved.
- Stir in marshmallows.
- Bring to boil, remove from heat.
- Add all chocolates.
- Stir until well blended.
- Add pecans.
- Pour into greased 9 X 13 glass dish.
- Cool, then refrigerate.
- In the cook time, I listed 10 minutes, it may take longer to boil.

197. The Delta Queen's Pralines Recipe

Serving: 2 | Prep: | Cook: 45mins | Ready in:

Ingredients

- 2 cups firmly packed dark brown sugar
- 2 cups granulated sugar
- 1/4 cup (1/2 stick) butter
- 1 cup evaporated milk
- 1 cup milk
- 1/4 teaspoon salt
- 1 1/2 teaspoons pure vanilla or maple extract (or a combination of both)
- 3 tablespoons light corn syrup
- 2 cups coarsely chopped pecans

Direction

- In a large, heavy saucepan, combine all the ingredients except the pecans and mix till well-blended. Cook, stirring, over moderate heat till the mixture registers 240 degrees F. on a candy thermometer or forms a soft ball when a glob is dropped into 1/2 cup cold water. Cool the mixture slightly, then beat with a wooden spoon till creamy. Add the pecans and stir till well blended and smooth. Drop the batter by the teaspoon onto waxed paper and let the pralines cool completely before serving or storing.
- Yield: About 3 1/2 dozen pralines

198. Toffee Recipe

Serving: 12 | Prep: | Cook: 12mins | Ready in:

Ingredients

- 3/4 c pecans, chopped
- 3/4 c brown sugar
- 1/2 c butter
- 1/2 c chocolate chips

Direction

- Butter 9x9x2 pan.
- Spread pecans in pan.
- Heat sugar and butter to boiling over medium low heat, stirring constantly, for 7 min.
- Immediately spread mixture evenly over nuts in pan.
- Sprinkle chocolate chips over hot mixture.
- Place baking sheet over pan so chocolate will melt.
- Spread melted chocolate over candy.
- Cut while hot.

- Chill until firm.

199. Traditional Buttermilk Pralines Recipe

Serving: 8 | Prep: | Cook: 20mins | Ready in:

Ingredients

- 2 cups sugar
- 1 cup buttermilk
- 2 tablespoons white corn syrup
- 1 teaspoon baking soda
- Pinch of salt
- Large lump of butter
- 1 teaspoon vanilla
- 1-1/2 cups pecans

Direction

- Combine sugar, buttermilk, corn syrup, baking soda and salt in a large sauce pan and boil until candy thermometer reading is 238 stirring frequently.
- Remove from heat then add butter, vanilla and pecans.
- Beat until right consistency to drop from spoon onto wax paper.
- It thickens quickly so work fast.

200. Trevor City Fudge Recipe

Serving: 0 | Prep: | Cook: 2hours | Ready in:

Ingredients

- 1 (14 oz) can sweetened condensed milk
- 3 cups peanut butter baking chips
- 1 tsp vanilla extract
- dash salt
- 1 cup M&M Plain candies ~or~ Reese's Pieces peanut butter candies
- 1/2 cup chopped pecans

Direction

- 1. Combine sweetened condensed milk and baking chips in a saucepan over boiling water (double boiler). Stir occasionally until chips are melted.
- 2. Take off of heat and add in flavouring, salt, candies and chopped nuts. Spoon into a buttered or foil lined 9x9-inch pan. Cool until firm.
- 3. Lift foil sling out of pan and onto a cutting board. Cut into 1" squares. Store covered at room temperature.

201. Triple Chocolate Sour Cherry Fudge Recipe

Serving: 60 | Prep: | Cook: 10mins | Ready in:

Ingredients

- 1 1/4 cups milk chocolate chips
- 1/2 cup plus 2 tablespoons evaporated milk
- 1/4 cup chocolate hazelnut spread (nutella)
- 1 teaspoon vanilla extract
- 1/4 teaspoon fine salt
- 1 (12-ounce) bag semisweet chocolate chips
- 1 1/2 cups dried sour cherries
- 3/4 cup roughly chopped pecans, toasted

Direction

- Line an 8- x 8-inch glass dish with foil; set aside.
- Put milk chocolate chips, evaporated milk, chocolate hazelnut spread, vanilla, salt and semisweet chocolate chips into a medium pot and cook over medium-low heat, stirring constantly, until smooth, about 5 minutes. Stir in cherries and pecans, then transfer mixture to prepared dish. Shake and tap dish gently on the countertop to remove any air bubbles from the fudge, then smooth out the top with the

back of a spoon. Cover and chill until set, about 3 hours.
- Loosen fudge from dish and turn out onto a cutting board; remove and discard foil. Using a serrated knife, cut fudge into pieces and serve.

202. Triple Nut Candy Recipe

Serving: 8 | Prep: | Cook: 35mins |Ready in:

Ingredients

- 1c. walnut halves
- 1c. pecan halves
- 1c brazil nuts,halved
- 1t. butter
- 1 1/2c sugar
- 1c heavy whipping cream
- 1/2c lt. corn syrup

Direction

- Place walnuts, pecans and Brazil nuts on a baking sheet. Bake at 350 for 8 mins or until toasted and golden brown; stirring once. Cool on wire rack.
- Line an 8" square pan with foil, grease the foil with butter and set aside
- In heavy saucepan, combine sugar, cream and corn syrup. Bring to a boil over med. heat, stirring constantly. Stir in toasted nuts. Cook, without stirring until a candy thermometer reads 238 degrees (soft ball stage). Remove from heat. Stir with a wooden spoon until creamy and thickened. Quickly spread into prepared pan; cool.
- Cover and refrigerate 8 hours or overnight. Using foil, lift candy out of pan; discard foil. Cut candy into squares. Store in airtight container in refrigerator. Makes 2 pounds.

203. Triple Nut Toffee Recipe

Serving: 36 | Prep: | Cook: 30mins |Ready in:

Ingredients

- 1/3c chopped pecans
- 1/3c slivered almonds
- 1/3c cahew halves and oieces
- 1/2c packed brown sugar
- 1/2c sugar
- 1c butter
- 1/4c water
- 1/2c semi-sweet chocolate morsels

Direction

- Heat oven to 350. Line jelly roll pan with foil. Spread nuts in pan. Bake uncovered 6 to10 mins, stirring occasionally, until light brown. Pour in small bowl; set aside. Set aside pan with foil to use in step 3.
- Meanwhile, in heavy 2qt. saucepan, cook sugars, butter and water over med-high heat 4 to 6 mins, stirring constantly with wooden spoon, until mixture comes to a full boil. Boil 20 to 25 mins, stirring frequently, until candy thermometer reaches 300 or small amount of mixture dropped into ice water forms a hard brittle strand.
- Stir in 1/2c of the nuts; immediately pour toffee into same foil-lined pan. Quickly spread mixture to 1/4" thickness with rubber spatula. Sprinkle with chocolate chips; let stand about 1 min or until chips are completely softened. Spread softened chocolate evenly over toffee. Sprinkle with remaining nuts.
- Refrigerate about 30 mins or until chocolate is firm. Break into pieces. Store in tightly covered container.

204. Turtle Squares Recipe

Serving: 40 | Prep: | Cook: 30mins |Ready in:

Ingredients

- 1 Tablespoon plus 1 cup butter (no substitutions), softened, divided
- 1-1/2 cups coarsely chopped pecans, toasted
- 1 to 1-1/2 cups chocolate chips (or part chocolate, part white)
- 2 cups packed brown sugar
- 1 cup light corn syrup
- 1/4 cup water
- 1 can (14 oz) sweetened condensed milk
- 2 teaspoons vanilla extract

Direction

- Line a 13 x 9 x 2 inch baking pan with foil. Butter the foil with one tablespoon of butter. Sprinkle with pecans and chips, set aside.
- In a heavy saucepan, over medium heat, melt remaining 1 cup butter. Add brown sugar, corn syrup and water.
- Cook and stir until mixture comes to a boil. Stir in milk.
- Cook, stirring constantly, until a candy thermometer reads 248 (firm ball stage).
- Remove from heat and mix in vanilla.
- Pour into prepared pan, do not scrape saucepan.
- Cool completely.
- Turn out onto a cutting board and peel off the foil. Cut into approximately 1 inch squares. Yields about 2-1/2 pounds. Store in a tightly sealed container in the refrigerator.

205. Turtles Recipe

Serving: 10 | Prep: | Cook: 30mins | Ready in:

Ingredients

- chocolate Base
- 1/2 cup cocoa powder
- 2 T.bls melted butter
- 2 Tbls coconut oil
- 1 t.eas vanilla
- 1/8 – 1/4 cup honey
- 3/4 cup pecans
- caramel sauce
- 1/4 cup heavy cream
- 1 cup maple syrup
- 1 tablespoon butter

Direction

- Chocolate
- Mix all ingredients.
- Spread onto a square pan approx. 1/8" thick or whatever you like.
- Sprinkle pecans on top of chocolate.
- Place in the freezer.
- Caramel
- Combine the cream, butter and maple syrup in the saucepan. Stir until well mixed.
- Cook over medium heat. You may gently swish sauce, but don't stir. Heat until temperature reaches 240° F 245° F, 10 to 15 minutes.
- Remove saucepan from the heat.
- Pour over pecans start in middle work to outer edge.
- Place back into freezer until firm.
- Cut into bite size pieces.
- Store in refrigerator.

206. Vanilla Fudge With Pecans Recipe

Serving: 12 | Prep: | Cook: 20mins | Ready in:

Ingredients

- 12 ounces white baking chocolate
- 8 ounces softened cream cheese
- 3 cups powdered sugar sifted
- 1 tablespoon vanilla extract
- 1/2 cup chopped pecans

Direction

- Melt chocolate as directed on package then beat cream cheese in large bowl with electric mixture until smooth then gradually beat in sugar on low speed until well blended.
- Add melted chocolate and vanilla and mix well.
- Stir in nuts.
- Spread evenly in foiled lined square pan.
- Garnish with additional nuts and refrigerate at least 1 hour.
- Cut into squares and store in refrigerator.

207. Wanda Riggs Fudge Recipe

Serving: 12 | Prep: | Cook: 20mins | Ready in:

Ingredients

- 4 cups sugar
- 1 large can evaporated milk
- 1 cube butter
- 1 jar marshmellow cream
- 32 oz Hersey Bars
- 3 cups pecans
- 1 teaspoon vanilla

Direction

- Bring sugar, milk and butter to a rolling boil. Boil 6 minutes stirring constantly.
- Take off stove. Add remaining ingredients.
- Stir until melted.
- Pour into 13 X 9-inch pan.

208. Whipped Fudge Recipe

Serving: 16 | Prep: | Cook: 15mins | Ready in:

Ingredients

- 1 Can (12 oz) evaporated milk
- 4 cups sugar
- 1.5 sticks of butter
- 1.5 bags of chocolate chips(or flavor of your choice)
- 1 tsp vanilla or (flavored extract of you choice-coconut, almond etc.)
- 1 cup of chopped nuts (your choice-walnuts, pecans, pistachios etc.)

Direction

- Bring evaporated milk, sugar and butter to a hard rolling boil on medium heat. I use a non-stick Dutch oven and a long handled wooden spoon. Boil for five minutes -stirring constantly so mixture does not BURN!
- Also, take a stick of butter around the rim of your Dutch over before cooking your milk/sugar/butter...Stops it from boiling over, plus it makes sure that all of the sugar gets incorporated...No grainy bits left in your mix!
- Now for the fun part!
- Chips, nuts, flavoring in large plastic bowl! Pour the hot mixture of milk/sugar/butter over the chips, nuts and flavoring.
- USE ELECTRIC HAND MIXER: Beat everything in the plastic bowl together on HIGH SPEED for Five Minutes. This will make the most incredibly light airy delicious decadent fudge you have ever had.
- NO MARSHMALLOW STICKY STUFF TO CLEAN UP!
- Whipping the fudge with the electric mixer eliminates the marshmallow-it's great but really is just more sugar and air. The mixer takes care of adding the air to your fudge. It's better for you as you are not adding more sugar. I also have added a large Hershey's candy bar-(broken into bits) with the chocolate chips for added richness. You can add any kind of bar you would like (white chocolate etc.
- Pour mixture into 9x13 greased pan. Spray or buttered, or wax paper lined.
- Let cool for at least 30 minutes. You can then cut it and turn it out if you want. I let this

fudge cool for at least another 4 hours to set up thoroughly.
- I have prepared this recipe using many different ingredients-it is fun to experiment and try new flavors together. Crushed candy canes, orange extract, almond extract and almonds, coconut, Maraschino cherries, cranberries, peanut butter and butterscotch, be brave, explore your options! My husband loves the peanut butter and milk chocolate chips together for this fudge.
- Happy Holidays and Enjoy...........DIANA!

209. White Bark Candy Recipe

Serving: 12 | Prep: | Cook: 6mins | Ready in:

Ingredients

- One package White or chocolate Bark
- 1 cup chopped pecans
- 1 cup chopped walnuts
- 1 8 oz package dried cranberries or orange flavored cranberries
- 1/2 - 1 teaspoon vanilla

Direction

- Chop the nuts, set aside.
- Tear off about 24 inches of waxed paper and having it laying so curl is down.
- Put all the cubes of bark in a microwave glass bowl. Plastic may work.
- Have a good glove to be able to hold the edge of the glass bowl it will be very hot when finally cooked. I just one of those total silicone gloves with 3 fingers and it worked well.
- Regardless of what the package says, it takes about 5 minutes in my 1000watt microwave to full melt all the cubes.
- After about 2 minutes, open the micro and stir the cubes a little, they should have a little melt going on.
- Stir after another minute, melting better, cubes getting smaller and getting a liquid.
- Cook another 30 seconds, stir. It is done when there are not any more cubes, pure liquid.
- Once it is melted, take from micro, place on counter and stir in vanilla and cranberries, stir well, coating the berries, dump in pecans, stir well, it will get thicker and harder to stir.
- Dump in walnuts and stir until coated, not is when you need that good bamboo stirring spoon.
- Careful pick up bowl, spoon out the goob of mix onto the wax paper and start spreading it out. You have to hold the paper with one hand the spread with the other using the spoon.
- Use the underside of the spoon to press the mix down to get it thinner and spread out, work it.
- Then comes the magic. Just let it set and soon it is very hard and you have this huge sheet. Break off pieces to serve, eat.
- I just recently added the walnuts, more crunch. First only used pecans. I need to cook the pecans and walnuts in the oven, I think it would bring out more of the nut flavor. If you try this, let me know how it turns out with the nuts bake first.
- A good Christmas treat. The bark is sometimes hard to find in the grocery store the closer to Christmas time.

210. White Chocolate And Eggnog Fudge Recipe

Serving: 0 | Prep: | Cook: 10mins | Ready in:

Ingredients

- Makes 2 dozen squares
- Ingredients:
- 1/2 cup butter
- 3/4 cup eggnog
- 2 cups sugar
- 1 1/4 cups (10 ounces) white chocolate bars, broken into pieces
- 1/2 teaspoon ground nutmeg

- 1 7 ounce jar marshmallow crème
- 1 cup chopped pecans
- 1 teaspoon rum or rum extract

Direction

- Directions:
- In a heavy saucepan, combine butter, eggnog, and sugar. Bring to a full rolling boil over medium-high heat, stirring constantly. Reduce heat to medium, and continue to boil, stirring frequently, 8 to 10 minutes or until mixture reaches 234°F (use candy thermometer).
- Remove from heat; add chocolate and nutmeg; stir until smooth. Add marshmallow crème, pecans and rum; mix well. Pour mixture into a 9-inch square pan lined with buttered foil. Cool completely; cut into 1 1/2-inch squares.
- Store in an airtight container in the refrigerator for up to one week.
- Microwave Instructions:
- In a 4-quart microwave-safe bowl, microwave butter on high for 1 minute or until melted. Add eggnog and sugar; mix well and microwave 6 minutes or until mixture comes to a rolling boil; stirring after 3 minutes.
- Scrape sides of bowl and mix well, continue microwaving 9 minutes more, scraping bowl and mixing after each 3 minutes, stir in chocolate until melted; continue as directed above.

211. White Chocolate Truffles Recipe

Serving: 30 | Prep: | Cook: 10mins | Ready in:

Ingredients

- 8 ounces white chocolate
- 48 pecan halves
- 6 tablespoons unsalted butter at room temperature
- 1-1/2 tablespoons water
- 1 large egg yolk

Direction

- Preheat oven to 300.
- Set aside a wax paper lined baking sheet.
- Chop white chocolate into small pieces and set aside.
- Toast nuts on a baking sheet in a single layer for 8 minutes then set them aside.
- In top of a double boiler over hot not boiling water melt chocolate and butter in the water.
- Stir until smooth then pour into a bowl and add the yolk.
- Continue beating until mixture is fluffy and cooled to room temperature.
- Chill for 4 hours then remove from refrigerator and form into 1" balls.
- Sandwich between 2 nut halves then chill until ready to serve.

212. White Fudge Recipe

Serving: 64 | Prep: | Cook: | Ready in:

Ingredients

- 2 - 3 ounce packages cream cheese, softened
- 1 6-ounce package white baking chocolate, melted
- 1 1/2 teaspoons vanilla extract
- Dash salt
- 5 cups powdered sugar unsifted
- 1 cup pecans, chopped (you can vary by using macadamia nuts)

Direction

- Generously butter an 8 x 8 x 2-inch baking pan.
- In a large mixer bowl at medium speed, beat cream cheese, white chocolate, vanilla and salt until well blended.
- At low speed, gradually add powdered sugar and beat until well blended and thick.
- Increase speed to medium and beat for 1 to 2 minutes or until fluffy.

- At low speed, beat in nuts.
- Spread evenly in prepared pan.
- Cover and refrigerate for 2 hours or until set.
- Cut into 1-inch pieces.
- Cover and store in the refrigerator up to 10 days.

213. White Popcorn Balls Recipe

Serving: 6 | Prep: | Cook: 10mins | Ready in:

Ingredients

- 1 cup granulated sugar
- 1/2 cup white corn syrup
- 1/2 cup water
- 2 tablespoons butter
- 1/2 tablespoon white vinegar
- 1/2 cup popped popcorn
- 1 cup pecans chopped and toasted

Direction

- Put sugar, corn syrup, water, butter and vinegar in a heavy saucepan.
- Cook to 260 on a candy thermometer.
- Pour over popped corn and toasted pecans then stir to coat.
- Butter hands and shape into balls.

214. White Or Chocolate Eggnog Fudge Recipe

Serving: 36 | Prep: | Cook: 15mins | Ready in:

Ingredients

- eggnog Fudge
- 1/2 cup sugar
- 3 cups miniature marshmallows
- 2/3 cup purchased eggnog
- 3 tablespoons butter
- 1 tablespoon corn syrup
- 1/8 teaspoon salt
- 1 cup (6 ounces) semisweet white chips or chocolate (your choice)
- 1 cup chopped pecans

Direction

- Butter sides of a heavy 3-quart saucepan. Add sugar, marshmallows, eggnog, butter, corn syrup, and salt to the saucepan; cook over low heat, stirring constantly, until sugar is dissolved. Turn heat up to medium and cook until mixture boils.
- Continue to cook, stirring constantly, to about 232°.
- Add chocolate chips and continue to cook for 5 minutes (should be at soft ball stage*), or until chocolate is melted. Stir in chopped nuts. Pour into a buttered 8-inch square pan. Cool to room temperature, then chill and cut into squares.
- Makes about 3 dozen pieces of eggnog fudge.
- *To Test for Soft Ball Stage
- A small amount of syrup dropped into chilled water forms a ball, but flattens when picked up with fingers (234° to 240°).

215. Wicked Kahlua Fudge Recipe

Serving: 64 | Prep: | Cook: 60mins | Ready in:

Ingredients

- 1-1/3 c. sugar
- 7 oz. marshmallow cream
- 2/3 c. evaporated milk
- 1/4 c. butter
- 1/4 c. Kahlua liquor
- 1/4 tsp. salt
- 2 c. semi-sweet chocolate chips
- 1 c. milk chocolate chips
- 1 c. chopped pecans or walnuts

- 1 tsp. EACH vanilla & Kahlua

Direction

- Line an 8" x 8" pan with foil.
- In a 3 qt. or little larger (it spits!) pan, bring to a boil the sugar, marshmallow, milk, butter, 1/4 c. Kahlua, & salt; boil FAST for 5 minutes while you keep stirring.
- Off heat, stir in chocolates till melted, then nuts, vanilla, and 1 tsp. Kahlua.
- Pour into foil and chill.
- Cut into squares to serve.

216. Yummy Buttermilk Candy Recipe

Serving: 16 | Prep: | Cook: 50mins | Ready in:

Ingredients

- 2 cups low-fat buttermilk
- 4 cups sugar
- 4 tablespoons butter, cut into 4 pieces
- 1-1/2 cups walnuts or pecans, chopped

Direction

- Line an 8 inch square pan baking pan with foil, leaving some excess over the sides. (You'll pull the fudge out with the excess later.) Grease the foil.
- Combine the sugar and buttermilk in a medium or large heavy-bottomed saucepan and bring to a boil over medium-high heat. (Be careful - buttermilk boils over in a hurry!)
- Reduce heat to low and simmer, stirring constantly, until the mixture reaches the soft-ball stage on a candy thermometer, 234-240 degrees. This will take 35-40 minutes. At this point, the mixture will be milky, yet translucent. And very, very hot.
- Off the heat, add the butter, mixing with a wooden spoon until the candy begins to thicken, about 5 minutes. Stir in the nuts until the mixture becomes difficult to stir, 3 minutes. Pour the mixture into the prepared pan and cool for at least 2 hours
- Remove and cut into 1-inch squares.
- The candy will store for 2 weeks.

217. Devinity Candy Recipe

Serving: 36 | Prep: | Cook: 20mins | Ready in:

Ingredients

- 3 cups sugar
- 3/4 cups light corn syrup
- pinch salt
- 3 egg whites, stiffly beaten
- 1 cup chopped pecans
- 3/4 tea vanilla 1
- 1 cup boiling water

Direction

- Bring sugar, water, syrup, and salt to a boil, boil 15 minutes. Pour mixture over stiffly beaten egg whites. Beat until it starts to thicken. Add vanilla and pecans.
- Beat until thick enough to drop a small amount at a time on wax paper. Cool. Yields about 36 pieces
- Grand ma says not too much, it will spoil your dinner

218. Microwave Pralines Recipe

Serving: 8 | Prep: | Cook: 6mins | Ready in:

Ingredients

- 1/3 cup evaporated milk
- 1 cup sugar
- 3/4 pecans
- 1 1/2 tablespoons butter

- 1 tsp. vanilla

Direction

- Mix all but vanilla extract in a 2 qt microwave safe bowl (I use glass measuring cup).
- Microwave on high for 6 minutes, stirring every 2 minutes.
- Add Vanilla and beat for a min. or 2, then quickly drop by teaspoonful onto wax paper.
- Allow to fully harden and cool before storing in airtight container.

219. Pecan Bark Recipe

Serving: 10 | Prep: | Cook: 10mins | Ready in:

Ingredients

- 1 cup unsalted butter, no substitutes
- 1 cup firmly packed brown sugar
- 1 cup chopped pecans
- 24 graham cracker squares

Direction

- Preheat oven to 350 degrees. Line a 10-by15- cookie sheet with aluminum foil. Lightly grease the foil. Place graham crackers on cookie sheet in one layer. (It should fit exactly 24.) Sprinkle pecans evenly over the top and set aside. Melt butter in a small saucepan. Add brown sugar, and stir until the mixture boils. Boil for 1 minute. Pour mixture evenly over graham crackers and pecans. Bake for 10 minutes. Remove from oven, and immediately place the hot cookie sheet in the freezer. Remove the pan after 1 hour, and break the bark into pieces. This candy does not need to be refrigerated.

220. Pina Coloda Bonbons Recipe

Serving: 36 | Prep: | Cook: 5mins | Ready in:

Ingredients

- 1 cup coconut
- 1/2 cup crushed pineapple, drained
- 1/2 cup chopped cherries
- 1/2 cup chopped pecans
- 1/2 to 3/4 cup sweetened condensed milk
- 1 bag milk chocolate chips

Direction

- Mix all fruit and milk together and refrigerate for 2 hours.
- Melt chocolate chips in a bowl starting with 1 minute, stir and then melt for 30 second intervals after that.
- Using chocolate molds, fill with melted chocolate to form shells and let set in fridge. Put about 1/4 to 1/2 tsp. filling in each and seal bottoms with more chocolate. Let set. Pop out of molds and enjoy.

221. Super Easy Cream Cheese Rum Fudge Recipe

Serving: 36 | Prep: | Cook: 1mins | Ready in:

Ingredients

- 2 3-ounce packages cream cheese, softened
- 2 tablespoons milk
- 4 cups sifted powdered sugar
- 1 teaspoon vanilla
- 1/2 to 1 teaspoon rum flavoring*
- 1-1/2 cups chopped walnuts or pecans
- 3 ounces unsweetened chocolate, melted and cooled

Direction

- 1. In a mixing bowl, combine softened cream cheese and milk. Gradually add the powdered sugar, beating the mixture until smooth.
- 2. Stir in 1 cup of the nuts, the vanilla, and rum flavoring. Stir in melted chocolate.
- 3. Immediately turn fudge mixture into a foil-lined, then buttered, 8x8x2-inch pan, pressing evenly into pan. Sprinkle with remaining nuts, pressing nuts lightly. Cover and chill for at least 1 hour before cutting into squares. Store the fudge in the refrigerator. Makes 36 pieces.
- Note
- Try substituting other flavors for rum, such as almond, peppermint, or orange extract.

222. Velveeta Cheese Fudge Recipe

Serving: 24 | Prep: | Cook: 10mins | Ready in:

Ingredients

- 8 ounces Velveeta cheese
- 8 tablespoons butter (1 stick)
- 2 pounds powdered sugar
- 1/4 cup cocoa
- 1 cups nuts (I use walnuts or pecans)
- 1 teaspoon vanilla

Direction

- Lightly butter 8x8 square pan
- Put sugar, cocoa, and nuts in large mixing bowl.
- Place cheese and butter in heavy sauce pan.
- Cook cheese and butter on low-medium heat until melted.
- Stir continuous to prevent burning.
- When completely melted, pour over sugar mixture. Add vanilla
- Stir all together until mixture is too thick; then use hands to completely mix.
- Put in pan. May need to blot the top to get rid of excess melted butter.
- Cut fudge when cooled and completely set.

Index

A
Almond 11
Apple 3,4,12,43
Apricot 3,21,35

B
Baking 65,76
Bran 3,9,12,24,41
Brazil nut 86
Butter 3,4,5,6,9,10,11,13,18,24,27,30,33,36,37,42,51,53,58,59,64,65,66,68,72,84,85,87,91,92

C
Caramel 3,4,5,13,14,15,18,43,44,54,59,60,68,73,87
Cashew 4,44,70
Cheese 3,5,16,20,28,93,94
Cherry 3,5,16,17,19,85
Chips 88
Chocolate 3,4,5,6,11,13,17,18,19,20,21,22,23,24,25,27,30,31,32,34,35,36,52,55,58,59,65,70,76,79,80,83,85,87,89,90,91
Cinnamon 4,42
Coconut 3,20,25,27
Crackers 3,18,19
Cranberry 3,26,27,28
Cream 3,4,5,20,24,28,29,30,41,58,62,72,73,93

D
Dark chocolate 75
Date 3,4,5,12,31,39,55,78

E
Egg 3,5,16,65,89,91

F
Fat 28,65,80
Fleur de sel 8
Flour 65
Fruit 3,11,27
Fudge 3,4,5,7,8,9,10,11,14,19,20,22,24,27,28,35,36,37,39,41,42,43,45,48,50,51,52,55,58,59,66,69,70,71,72,73,75,77,78,79,80,84,85,87,88,89,90,91,93,94

G
Gin 5,73

H
Honey 4,31,42

J
Jelly 58
Jus 22,47,49,89

M
Macadamia 4,42,44
Macaroon 3,35
Margarine 75
Marshmallow 3,4,29,36,38,46,75
Milk 73,75
Molasses 4,63

N
Nut 3,4,5,11,15,16,23,27,28,33,36,37,41,42,46,54,65,70,79,80,81,82,86

O
Orange 3,4,30,47,55,56

P

Pear 5,73

Pecan 1,3,4,5,6,9,10,12,22,23,24,25,30,42,45,49,51,52,56,59,60,62,63,64,65,67,68,75,76,78,81,82,87,93

Peel 11

Pepper 3,5,34,71

Pie 4,58,65,69,76,85

Pistachio 3,5,19,72

Popcorn 5,91

Port 33

Praline 3,4,5,10,30,34,36,42,44,47,48,54,64,67,68,83,84,85,92

Pumpkin 4,5,66,69,79

R

Raisins 75

Rice 17

Rum 5,74,75,93

S

Salt 3,5,6,76

Soda 65

Sugar 4,5,44,49,51,55,65,68,75,79,80

T

Tangerine 5,72

Tea 63,89

Toffee 3,4,5,18,23,33,37,38,39,49,52,76,84,86

Truffle 3,4,5,17,23,25,46,78,90

Conclusion

Thank you again for downloading this book!

I hope you enjoyed reading about my book!

If you enjoyed this book, please take the time to share your thoughts and post a review on Amazon. It'd be greatly appreciated!

Write me an honest review about the book – I truly value your opinion and thoughts and I will incorporate them into my next book, which is already underway.

Thank you!

If you have any questions, **feel free to contact at:** author@papayarecipes.com

Cindy Taylor

papayarecipes.com

Made in the USA
Columbia, SC
03 April 2025